Lecture Notes

Anatomy and Physiology For the Respiratory Therapist

Peter A. Petroff, MD

2019 update

I want to thank Dr. Gregg Marshall, Dr. Chris Russian and Dr. Nicholas Henry for their encouragement in this project. I want to also thank Elizabeth Rodriquez, for helping to edit the manuscript.

Lecture Notes is dedicated to all the students I have taught over the last forty years at Texas State University. They are my inspiration.

Index

Part One

Lecture One	Introduction	1
Lecture Two	Blood	11
Lecture Three	Anatomy and Physiology of the Heart	23
Lecture Four	The Electrocardiogram	33
Lecture Five	Common Heart Disorders	46
Lecture Six	The Circulation	56
Lecture Seven	The Upper Airways	66
Lecture Eight	The Thorax	75

Part Two

Lecture Nine	The Lower Airways	86
Lecture Ten	Static Properties of the Lungs	92
Lecture Eleven	Dynamic Properties of the Lung	100
Lecture Twelve	Ventilation Perfusion Relationships	105
Lecture Thirteen	Diffusion	110
Lecture Fourteen	Pulmonary Function Testing	116
Lecture Fifteen	Control of Ventilation	127

Part Three

Lecture Sixteen	Diseases of the Airways	134
Lecture Seventeen	Restrictive Disease	149
Lecture Eighteen	Sleep and Sleep Disorders	164
Lecture Nineteen	The Kidney	179
Lecture Twenty	Fetal development and Aging	190
Lecture Twenty-one	Exercise, diving and high altitude	198
Lecture Twenty-two	The Immune System	206

INDEX	214

Copyright 2019

Lecture One

Introduction

None of us, not even Respiratory Therapists, think about our lungs very much. We don't walk about thinking, "Inhale! Exhale! Inhale! Exhale!" When we hurry because we're late for class we don't say, "Breathe faster! Breathe deeper!" And when we sleep we don't say, "Slow down! Relax! Breathe slower!"

Breathing just happens. But why do we need to breathe at all? Is it just a bad habit we should all try to give up, like ice cream? A respiratory therapist might say, "It's because we need oxygen! We can't live without oxygen! Everybody knows that!"

But if oxygen is the answer, why is it the answer? After all, there are trillions of creatures, some of them actually living inside us, that don't need oxygen at all.

In order to understand the role of oxygen and our apparent need for it, we must travel back eons of years. Our world was formed about 4,000,000,000 years ago. It was hot, wet, and crammed with toxic chemicals. Some of the chemicals could burn the paint off your car! Gradually, according to some scientists, atoms combined into larger and larger chemicals which somehow became able to reproduce themselves. Over a period of billions of years or so the first life-forms appeared and evolution began. Other scientists think that life-forms travelled as passengers on asteroids from the deepest space, space so hot and radioactive that chemical activity was constant and had gone on for even more billions of years. These asteroids brought with them early alien life-forms which, when the asteroid crashed into earth, took hold and began to evolve into life as we know it.

Either way, and I prefer the asteroid theory myself, these chemicals ultimately formed active and reproducing complex chemicals. At first they slushed freely about in the great seas. Then they developed walls or envelopes to protect themselves from other chemicals floating free in the sea. Slowly, after many millions of years, the first cell was born.

The first cells were simple. They had an envelope or cell wall for protection, some chemicals for reproduction, and some chemicals for manufacturing all the other chemicals they needed for replacement parts. For most of these cells, oxygen was not required and there probably would not have been a lot of it about in the great sea anyway.

Nowadays, a typical cell consists of a nucleus with reproductive chemicals, either Deoxyribonucleic Acid (DNA) or Ribonucleic Acid (RNA) encased by the nuclear membrane, a surrounding cytoplasm, also called the *Cytosol,* which is then bounded by a dense cell wall. There are several organelles (small organs) in the cytoplasm. Each has their own highly specialized function.

The *Mitochondria* are the power plants. Chemicals, such as sugars, fats, and amino acids are broken down to make the energy needed by the cell for all its function. Interestingly in humans at least, the *Mitochondria* also has DNA, just like the nucleus. But the *Mitochondrial* DNA is inherited only from the mother because the ova contain mitochondria but not the sperm.

The *Ribosomes* are the organelles which function to make the large proteins needed for the cell's infrastructure such as the cell wall. The ribosomes also make different types of proteins including the enzymes which catalyze or enhance the chemical reactions in the cell.

The *Lysosomes* contain the enzymes which break down and recycle waste material, perhaps damaged bits of the intracellular superhighway or a broken cell wall.

The *Endoplasmic Reticulum* is the superhighway that allows the rapid transfer of chemicals from the nucleus to the organelles and to the cell wall.

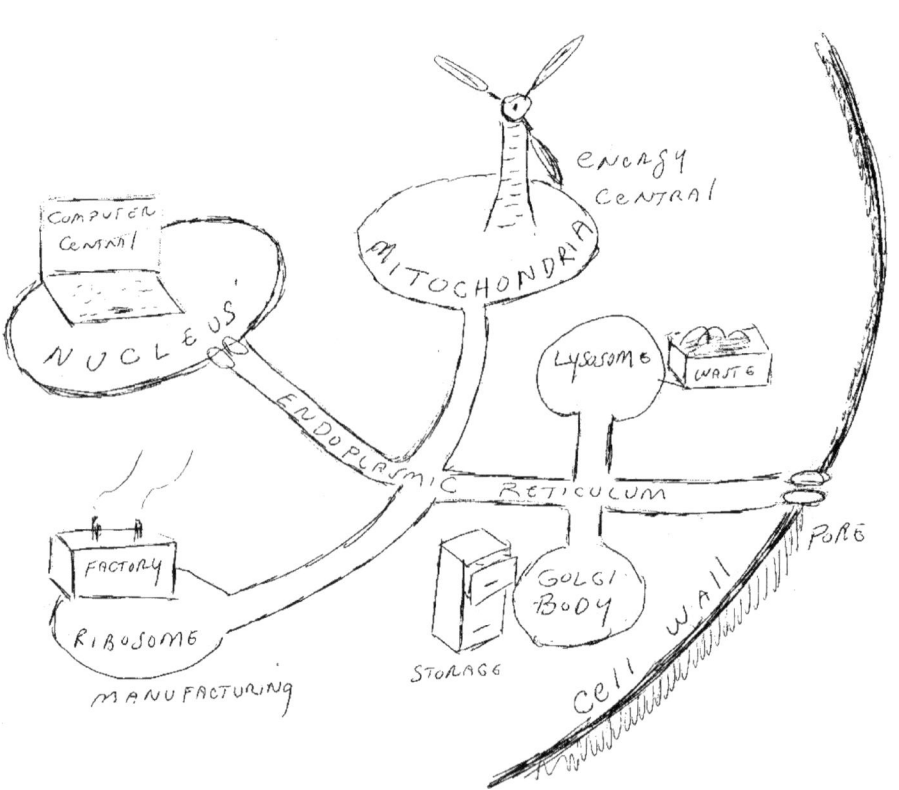

The Typical Cell

All along the *Endoplasmic Reticulum* are large extrusions where the cell's waste material can be collected for disposal. The large sacs are called *Golgi Apparati*. The waste is collected in these sacs and transported to the cell wall. When the sacs reach the cell boundary they merge with the cell wall and then whisk their contents out of the cell.

Even the cell wall has several functions in addition to protecting the cell from its environment. The cell wall consists of layers of glycoproteins and lipids. There are pores in the cell wall which can open and close. These pores are for the transport of chemicals needed for energy such as amino acids and sugars as well as the transport of electrolytes such as calcium, magnesium, potassium and sodium.

The cell requires a lot of energy. It needs energy to reproduce itself, energy for building and breaking down proteins and sugars, energy for transporting chemicals along the *endothelial reticulum*, and energy for opening and closing the pores of the cell wall.

But the energy needed for these activities is not oxygen.

Metabolism

To get a foothold on what the source of the cell energy really is, we must understand a little basic chemistry. Yes, even Respiratory Therapists need to know a little chemistry. We might as well bite our lip and dive right in.

We will start at the basic level, the atom. Then we will discuss bonding between atoms. Finally we will look at the most important chemicals found in our bodies.

Even the simplest atom, hydrogen, contains a proton, neutron, and an electron. The proton has a single positive charge, the neutron has no charge at all, and the electron has a negative charge. But, like all of life, it is not quite that simple.

The nucleus of the atom is composed of protons and neutrons. The proton and neutron are made up of *Quarks,* which turn out to be the basic building blocks of nature. The proton is made up of two "Up" quarks and one "Down" quark. The neutron is made up of two "Down" quarks and one "Up" quark. The "Up" quarks have 2/3rds positive charge and "Down" quarks have 1/3 negative charge. But the weight of the three quarks makes up only 1% of the weight of either a proton or neutron. 99% of the weight is energy!

The electron used to be thought of as a particle which flies around the nucleus. While the electron is a particle, it is also something more. It is an electrical charge which forms a cloud surrounding the nucleus. Thus the electron can be both a particle and a wave at the same time!

The bigger the atom, the more levels of electron clouds it has. For example, the helium atom has two protons, two neutrons, and two electrons. The two electrons are happy to occupy the cloud closest to the nucleus. However, lithium has a nucleus with three protons and three (or four) neutrons. It also has three electrons but since the inner cloud can only handle two electrons, the third electron orbits the nucleus in a cloud further away from the nucleus. Thus lithium has two levels of clouds.

The cloud nearest the nucleus can take only two electrons, the next cloud can take eight electrons as can the third. The fourth can take up to sixteen electrons. The bigger the atom the more clouds there are and the more unstable the molecule will be. If a cloud can handle eight electrons but has only one, it can either share that one electron with another atom or borrow up to seven electrons from another atom. Thus lithium, with one electron in its outermost chain, can share its electron with chlorine which has a total of 17 electrons. Lithium, by giving its electron, has a positive charge of one. Chlorine has two electrons in its innermost ring and eight electrons in its middle ring. Both rings are full. But its outermost ring has only seven electrons and that ring can take eight. Chlorine can share an electron with lithium which has only one electron in its outer ring. They will form the molecule lithium chloride. They are truly made for each other. A marriage made in heaven. The bond, called an *Ionic Bond,* will be quite tight as neither atom will want to give away the shared electron away. This is the strongest form of bonding. To break this type of bond will require a lot of energy and when you finally break this bond there will be a whole lot of energy released.

Another example is water itself, which, of course, is H_2O. We have already discussed Hydrogen. Oxygen has eight protons and neutrons. Thus, it must also have eight electrons. The inner ring has two and is full. The outer ring has only six electrons and thus has space for two more. Thus two hydrogens can each donate their single electron to fill oxygen's outermost ring. This is also an ionic bond.

But this is not the only type of bond.

Two positive or two negative atoms can bond together. For example Hydrogen has only one electron in its cloud. Thus two Hydrogen atoms can get together and share their electron thus filling their cloud. When two atoms of similar charge bind together the bond is called a *Covalent Bond*. While the electrons are happy to share a ring, the positively charged Hydrogen nuclei don't like being that close together. Just try putting the north poles of two magnets together. Just won't happen. The repulsion weakens the bond. The bond is easier to break and produces less energy when it does break.

The last type of bond is called the *Van Der Waals Bond*. This bonding occurs because molecules like water aren't straight like we name them. Water is H_2O, two atoms of Hydrogen joined to one atom of oxygen. In reality water looks like this:

(+)

H H

O

(-)

The two hydrogens are on the top of the water molecule and the oxygen is on the bottom. The Hydrogen side has a relative positive charge and the oxygen a relative negative charge. Thus this "neutral" molecule actually has a positive side and a negative charge. Thus two water molecules can line up. The negative sides are attracted to the positive sides. The bonds that form are very weak and thus produce little energy when they are broken apart. But this is one of the commonest bonds we will deal with when we begin to discuss Hemoglobin, oxygen, and carbon dioxide.

Now that we know all there is to know about atoms and the types of bonds holding them together we can finally deal with the chemicals that make up our cells.

Water

Water is ubiquitous. It makes up 70% of the human body. Most of the water is "intracellular"; it is located inside the cell.

In the simplest cells water functions mainly as a solvent for the electrolytes, sugars and proteins that romp about the cytosol. Because of its polar nature, it is the universal solvent. Any chemical that carries a charge will dissolve in water. They are called "hydrophilic" or water-loving. On the other hand fats, which don't have a charge, won't be able to dissolve in water. They are "hydrophobic".

The water molecule doesn't have a charge; it is neutral. But because of its V like shape it has a positive side and a negative side. More importantly water can break down into a hydrogen ion (H+) and a hydroxyl group (OH-).

Proteins

Proteins are large molecules that are made up of *amino acids*. Amino Acids must contain both an "amino" group and an "acid" group. The "amino" group is made up of a nitrogen atom and two hydrogen Atoms or NH_2. An atom of nitrogen has 7 protons and neutrons and thus has seven electrons. The inner ring of electrons is full but the outer ring has only five electrons. Thus there is space for three more electrons and, therefore, NH2 still has one free binding site. In an amino acid, the NH_2 binds to a carbon atom. Still because of the shape of the "amino" group, it can <u>accept</u> yet another hydrogen and become positively charged.

The "acid" group is much more complex. It consists of a carbon atom bound to an oxygen molecule and a hydroxyl group, which is made up of one oxygen bound to a hydrogen. Thus it looks like COOH. Carbon has six protons, six neutrons and six electrons. The inner ring is full but here are only four electrons in its outer ring. Thus it can accept up to four more electrons. The oxygen can give two, and the hydroxyl group (OH) can give one. Thus, there is one free space which, in an amino acid, is another Carbon atom. The COOH radical is able to <u>donate</u> the hydrogen and is thus an acid.

Thus, the structure of an amino acid is:

$$+ NH_3 \text{—Carbon Chain—} COO -$$

The amino side is relatively positive, the acid side is relatively negative. Therefore, long chains of amino acids can be formed using Van der Waals binding.

Proteins are the structural backbone of all the tissues. In addition, enzymes, hemoglobin, hormones and antibodies are all proteins.

Carbohydrates

Carbohydrates are "sugars". They are easily recognized since all the sugars end in "ose" like lactose, sucrose, galactose, and so on. Chemically they are made up of rings of carbon atoms, each carbon atom having a hydrogen and a hydroxyl (OH) group. Thus the formula for a sugar is always:

$$C_n (H_2O)_n$$

Glucose, a six carbon sugar, is: "$C_6 \ H_{12} \ O_6$"

GLUCOSE

A quick glance at the molecule shows the large number of ionic bonds between carbon and the hydroxyl group present in a sugar molecule, making it a great choice for both the storage and the production of energy. The bonds between the carbon and hydrogen are covalent bonds which are not as rich in energy however.

Ribose is a five carbon sugar. It forms the basis of both DNA and RNA:

RIBOSE

Carbohydrates can also combine with proteins to form "glycoproteins" which are the building blocks of the cell wall and other structures.

Where do sugars come from? Carbohydrates are created by plants. 6 CO_2 molecules and six H_2O molecules are combined to form $C_6 H_{12} O_6$ in the presence of chlorophyll. Thus plants are extremely important in removing carbon dioxide from our atmosphere. The simple sugars in plants are chained together to form the complex sugar cellulose.

Lipids

Lipids consists of very long, I mean very long carbon chains. The two free bonds on each carbon are shared with a hydrogen atom. If the lipid has a COO- radical at one end it is called a fatty acid. Three fatty acid chains can combine with a "glycerol" molecule to make up a fat. Because the molecules are mostly carbon and hydrogen they don't have a lot of sites for interactions with other chemicals and are essentially insoluble in water, which as we said earlier, is relatively charged.

Fats are made up of fatty acids which have a long, hydrophobic ("just don't like water"), chain of carbons filled with covalent hydrogen bonds, but ending in a hydrophilic (just loves water), acid-like structure ($COO^- H^+$). It is an acid because the hydrogen can split away or be shared.

FATTY ACID

Long chained hydrocarbon with an acid ending

Most fats exist bound to glycerol. Three fatty acids are bound to one three-carbon sugar molecule called glycerol. The glycerol molecule shares its oxygen electrons with the fatty acids. One end of the fat, the fatty chain part, is very hydrophobic but one end, the glycerol end, is hydrophilic.

TYPICAL FAT

The lipids form part of the cell wall along with the glycoproteins. The lipid hydrophobic end protects the inside of the cell from water and charged particles. The hydrophilic ends bind to each other and to the glycoproteins. The glycoproteins form the pores in the cell wall.

Lipids can also be made into ring-like structures such as "steroids" which include cholesterol and cortisone as wells chemicals like Arachidonic Acid which is metabolized into the leukotrienes and prostaglandins. These are all fatty acids which are important in the "inflammatory pathway".

Nucleotides

The last chemicals we must deal with are the nucleotides. A nucleotide is made up of a ringed compound containing the nitrogen atom, bound to a five carbon sugar, either Ribose or deoxyribose, which is bound to at least one phosphate group (PO4). The nucleotides form the basic structure of DNA and RNA.

Even more important the nucleotide, **Adenosine Triphosphate**, is <u>the most important chemical in our body</u>. It is the source of all the energy our bodies use in movement, thinking, breathing, dancing, and whatever else we do.

Adenosine triphosphate consists of adenosine bound to ribose which is then bound to a chain of three phosphate molecules. Each phosphate group is made up of a phosphorus atom attached to three oxygen molecules all of which are ionic bonds. One glance at the molecule shows just how much energy is available.

$$\text{Adenosine} - \text{Ribose} - \text{Phosphate} = \text{phosphate} = \text{phosphate}$$

(The = represents very high energy ionic bonds.)

We use more than 140 pounds of ATP a day even though at any given moment there are only about 0.1 pounds present in our bodies. Each molecule is recycled 1400 times a day. ATP opens and closes the pores on the cell wall for transport of electrolytes, water, sugar, and other chemicals. It energizes the synthesis of DNA, proteins, lipids, and complex sugars. It makes the high energy creatinine phosphate which powers our muscles. It powers our brain cells. It even is the power supply for the light of a firefly.

Energy is produced from the ATP when it is broken down into adenosine monophosphate (only one phosphate) and pyrophosphate (two phosphates bound together):

ATP > AMP + P = P + energy

The P = P is known as pyrophosphate

ATP is especially important to us as Respiratory Therapists because ATP can be metabolized into Cyclic AMP. This reaction is catalyzed by the enzyme *Adenyl Cyclase*. Cyclic AMP is the chemical which causes our airways to dilate. We will discuss this reaction a lot more in the section on Asthma.

Oxygen

If ATP is the source of all our energy, why do we need oxygen at all?

Oxygen was discovered by Antoine Lavoisier in 1787. Within forty years, it was clear that oxygen was needed for life as we know it. But why?

ATP is produced in the mitochondria from the breakdown of glucose. The initial phase, called *glycolysis* does not require oxygen at all. In this reaction Glucose, a six carbon sugar, is split into two pyruvate molecules, each having three carbons. Two ATP's are required to energize the reaction but four ATP's are produced. Only two percent of the energy present in a molecule of sugar is released. Not enough energy is made for us to operate but perhaps enough is made for a simple cell living in the great sea. Worse still, the pyruvate molecule may be converted to lactic acid.

Oxygen is required in order for the pyruvate to be metabolized, or broken down further. This second phase is called the *Krebs Cycle* and *Electron Transport System*. The second phase produces 30% of the energy in a molecule of glucose and is carried out entirely in the mitochondria. Amino acids and fatty acids can also enter the pathway and thus, like glucose, can be used to make ATP's.

The reactions turn the glucose molecule into Carbon Dioxide and Water:

$$C_6 H_{12} O_6 > 6 \, CO2 + 6 \, H_2O + 36 \, ATP's$$

Thus when oxygen is present, the glucose can be metabolized by the Krebs Cycle, and eighteen times more energy can be released from the glucose molecule. However, oxygen is consumed and carbon dioxide is released. The cell must have a mechanism for securing oxygen and releasing carbon dioxide. Otherwise the carbon dioxide will build up to very high and poisonous levels.

If you are a tiny creature made up of a handful of cells living in the great sea this certainly is not a problem. Oxygen can diffuse in and carbon dioxide diffuse out through the porous cell wall. But if you are a bird, fish, or mammal you need to develop a complex system to accomplish this feat.

We call the transfer of oxygen and carbon dioxide "*Respiration*". All creatures respire but only creatures with lungs breathe. We shouldn't really talk about the respiratory rate; we should talk about the breathing rate or "rate of breathing".

Now What About FISH

Do fish breathe? Certainly NOT in the sense that we do. They don't have any lungs. But they have gills, which, like the lungs, are devices to transfer oxygen and carbon dioxide to and from the fish's cells. The gills consist of myriads of tiny capillaries which are separated from the sea water by a thin membrane. Gases can easily diffuse (transfer) across this tiny membrane.

Thus in one sense, fishes don't breathe. Instead they gulp water and force it through the gills. They have to gulp a lot of water.

Can human beings breathe under water? Can our lungs work just like the gills of a fish?

A liter of air has 210 cubic centimeters of oxygen while a liter of water has only 8 cubic centimeters. Oxygen diffuses 10,000 times faster in air than in water. Water is 100 times more viscous and 777 times denser than air. Thus the gills have to be extremely efficient in order to perform gas exchange.

We require 250 cc of oxygen a minute. Thus if we had gills, we would have to gulp down 33 liters of water a minute! That would require a lot of energy and leave very little time for speaking or eating.

With few exceptions, gills only work in water. The dense water is required to keep the gills open. When a fish is taken out of water the gills collapse and the fish dies.

Thus, unless you are Esther Williams who spent her entire Hollywood career in swimming pools, you are better off with lungs

Finally, in order to take advantage of either gills or lungs, the body had to evolve a complex system which includes, not only the lungs and gills, but also a muscular system to bring air or water into contact with the capillaries of the gills and lungs, a circulatory system to transport the gases from the gills or lungs to the rest of the body and a pump to operate the circulatory system. There also had to be an efficient way of carrying the gases in the circulatory system.

This course is all about the blood, heart, the circulatory system and, of course, the lungs. We will discuss how they work and what can go wrong with them.

Lastly we will study, how the systems develop and how exercise, sleep, and high altitude can affect them.

IMPORTANT CONCEPTS TO REMEMBER FROM THIS LECTURE

1. What are the types of bonding found in chemicals?

    — Ionic, covalent, and Van der Waals

2. ATP is composed of:

    — Adenosine, ribose, and three phosphate ions two of them containing high energy bonding (ionic)

3. When oxygen is present, how much more ATP can be produced?

    — 18 times more (36 versus 2 molecules of ATP)

Lecture Two

Blood

What is blood? Is it:

1. The red stuff that oozes out of a beautifully prepared cut of beef tenderloin at Chez Paul's fine restaurant?
2. The stuff that oozes out of the knife wounds inflicted on a movie heroine while she showers?
3. A type of superhighway, carrying information from one part of the body to another?

The red stuff from a cut steak is red dye. A fine aged steak looks like beef jerky. The stuff oozing out of the heroine's knife wounds in Alfred Hitchcock's great movie *Psycho* was chocolate milk.

That leaves as our only choice, 'a type of superhighway'. One of the functions of blood which we won't spend much time on, unfortunately, is the transport of hormones from one organ to another. The pancreas makes Insulin and Glucagon which must reach the liver and muscles in order to control our sugar. The pituitary gland makes Growth Hormone which must travel to the bone and other structures to allow us to grow. The thyroid gland makes Thyroxine which must be transported to all the tissues of our body in order to regulate our metabolism. Our blood is a conduit for all these hormones and many, many more.

But blood is far more than that. Blood is also a solvent carrying dissolved electrolytes such as Sodium, Potassium, Calcium, Chloride, as well as chemicals such as sugar and amino acids needed for energy and growth, and more complex ions such as bicarbonate, all of which are needed by the cells of the body.

Most important for us, the blood carries oxygen and carbon dioxide. It carries oxygen from the lungs to the tissues and carbon dioxide from the tissues to the lungs.

The blood also carries cells including the Red Blood Cell or RBC, the White Blood Cells or WBC, and a cell fragment called a Platelet. Each has a specific purpose and a specific history.

Plasma versus Serum

One cause of confusion in a discussion of blood is, "What is the difference between *plasma* and *serum?*" Are they the same?

No, *Plasma* is the clear yellow part of the blood which is found after the cellular components have been removed by centrifugation. *Serum* goes one step further. It is the fluid from which the proteins such as fibrinogen, important in clotting, have also been removed. Plasma will clot; serum, because it does not have any clotting factors present, will not.

We can get a sample of *Plasma* by simply standing a tube of blood upright in a rack. The cellular components of the blood will drop to the bottom and a yellowish fluid will remain at the top some of which will clot. The yellowish fluid is the plasma. Plasma is used to rehydrate patients because it can still clot.

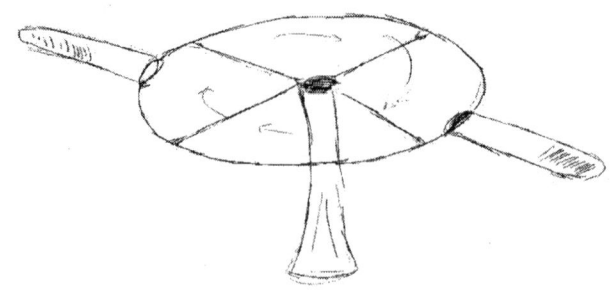

A SIMPLE CENTRIFUGE:

AS THE TUBES SPIN AROUND THE CENTRAL CORE,

THE CENTRIFUGAL FORCE PUSHES THE HEAVIER MATERIAL

TO THE BOTTOM OF THE TUBE.

In order to make *Serum,* the sample of blood is placed in a tube and spun in a centrifuge. The heavier parts of the sample, containing the red blood cells, white blood cells, and platelets, will be forced to the bottom of the tube as will the fibrinogen involved in clotting. The serum, which is much lighter, will remain at the top and can be siphoned off. Serum is used for diagnostic testing such as measuring the Sodium, Potassium and Calcium in the blood. It is also used to measure the levels of certain drugs such as Theophylline, a drug used in treating asthma.

Plasma is the crude product resulting from the precipitation of blood while serum is the plasma less the fibrinogen and other clotting factors.

Blood contains both the formed elements and plasma.

Blood makes up about eight percent of our body mass. Thus men have about five liters of blood while women have about four liters of blood. Three quarters of the blood is found in the circulation with most of that in the veins. 15% of the blood is found in the lungs and 10% in the heart.

The Red Blood Cell

The Red Blood Cell or RBC is the main cellular component of the blood, making up about 45% of blood. Unlike other cells, the RBC doesn't have a nucleus. Nor does the RBC have mitochondria or endoplasmic reticulum. But the RBC is still metabolically active and is able to produce ATP's from chemicals found in its cytosol or cytoplasm.

The shape of the RBC is unique among cells. It is a biconcave disc packed with hemoglobin, the iron-containing protein that transports oxygen.

The RBC's are formed in the bone marrow and are derived from the hematopoietic stem cells. The hormone, *Erythropoietin,* which is secreted by the kidneys in response to hypoxemia, which means *low oxygen in the blood,* is the driving force for the production of the RBC. The RBC measures about 7 to 8 micra in diameter but because the young RBC is pliable it can squeeze through capillaries that measure only 6 micra across. As the RBC ages, it becomes much less pliable and after about 120 days it is removed by the spleen and its chemical components recycled.

The production of hemoglobin, which makes up more than a third of the RBC, requires three common minerals and vitamins: Iron, Vitamin B12, and Folic Acid.

The *Hematocrit* is the portion of the blood made up by the RBC's. It is measured by centrifuging a sample of blood in a tube and seeing what percentage of the blood is made up of the RBC's. Thus the *Hematocrit* is expressed as a percentage. The normal value is about 45%

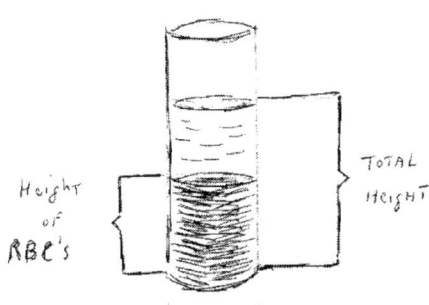

The hematocrit = the height of the RBC's divided by the total height.

A TEST TUBE AFTER CENTRIFUGATION

THE RBC'S FORM THE RED AT THE BOTTOM OF THE TUBE. ABOVE THEM IS A TINY WHITE BAND OF WHITE BLOOD CELLS AND ABOVE THEM IS THE SERUM.

On the other hand, the *Hemoglobin concentration* is the amount of hemoglobin present in 100 centiliters (100 milliliters) of blood measured in grams. A hemoglobin of 12 means that there are 12 grams of hemoglobin in 100 centiliters of blood. The hemoglobin concentration is very important when we discuss how much oxygen blood can carry.

While both the hematocrit and hemoglobin concentration are important, the hemoglobin concentration is most important for respiratory physiology since it is the hemoglobin which transports oxygen.

Patients can either have the right amount of RBC's, "too few" RBC's, or "too many" RBC's. "Too few" RBC's is called *anemia*. "Too many" is called *polycythemia*.

Anemia has many causes. The most common cause is, of course, blood loss and is most often seen in young women who have very heavy menses or patients who have had extensive surgery.

Anemia can be caused by iron deficiency. Iron is a mineral required for the production of hemoglobin. The RBC's in a patient deficient of iron will be small or *microcytic*, and have less hemoglobin.

Anemia can also be caused by deficiencies of Vitamin B12 and Folic Acid. The RBC's in these cases will be large or *macrocytic*.

Certain blood cancers such as leukemia or multiple myeloma cause anemia as well as can renal or kidney failure.

Polycythemia can be primary, due to a problem with the bone marrow itself which is called *Polycythemia Vera* ("True Polycythemia"), or secondary, due to hypoxemia. The kidneys of a patient with hypoxemia will produce a lot of erythropoietin which will force the bone marrow to produce a lot of RBC's. Secondary polycythemia can also be seen in a patient who has lost his spleen. The spleen is the major organ for the breakdown of the RBC. If it is absent, usually due to surgery following abdominal trauma, the RBC's will remain in the blood longer.

The most important function of the RBC is to carry oxygen from the lungs to the tissues. Oxygen can be dissolved in blood but the amount of oxygen that can be dissolved is very small. The amount of dissolved oxygen is related to the partial pressure of the oxygen in the blood.

Dissolved oxygen in cc/100 cc of blood = .003 X pO_2

Thus, if the pO_2 is 80, the amount of oxygen dissolved in the blood is .24 cc per 100 cc of blood

Even if the patient is breathing pure oxygen, his pO_2 will be only about 570 and the amount of dissolved Oxygen will be 1.7 cc per 100 cc of blood. But we need to carry about 20 cc of oxygen per 100 cc of blood in order to function at our best. With less than 1 cc of Oxygen per 100 cc of blood the heart would have to pump 20 times as fast. Instead of a heart rate of 70 we would have a heart rate of 1400. Our heart doesn't even beat that fast when we fall in love.

It is clear from the equation that dissolved oxygen is just not very efficient of effective.

But insects, reptiles, birds, fishes, and mammals have all developed a second way of transporting the oxygen. All these creatures use a large protein called *hemoglobin* to transport the oxygen. The hemoglobin molecule differs from species to species and there are even several types of hemoglobin in humans. There is a hemoglobin F, seen in fetuses and young infants, as well as hemoglobin S, seen in patients with Sickle Cell Disease, and Hemoglobin A, which is found in most adults.

The large hemoglobin protein is made up of four amino acid chains: two alpha chains and two beta chains. Each chain contains a molecule of iron (Fe) bound by nitrogen atoms into a *heme* molecule which sits in the center of each chain. Each iron atom can bind one molecule of O_2. Thus each hemoglobin molecule can bind up to four molecules of oxygen. In fact, one gram of hemoglobin can bind 1.34 grams of oxygen. Thus if your hemoglobin concentration is 15 gm's/100 cc of blood you can carry 15 X 1.34 or 20.1 gm's of hemoglobin in every 100 cc of your blood. That is a lot more oxygen than is dissolved in your blood.

The hemoglobin system is more complicated than that. The amount of oxygen bound to the hemoglobin is related to the Oxygen Saturationwhich is not related **directly** to the partial pressure of oxygen as you would expect.

This occurs because of the nature of the hemoglobin molecule. It is very difficult to bind the first oxygen onto the hemoglobin molecule, but once that first oxygen is bound, it is easier to attach the second and even easier to attach the third. Thus we get the S shaped SaO_2/PaO_2 curve.

The most important "factoids" we need to remember is that at a PaO_2 of 60 torr, the Oxygen Saturation is about 90%.

Why would we want the curve to be shaped like an S? In the lungs the PaO_2 is very high so the hemoglobin becomes saturated. On the other hand, because of the S shaped curve Oxygen can be released from the blood into the tissues a lot easier as the pO2 falls. In the tissues the PaO_2 is much lower and it is easier for the oxygen to leave the hemoglobin and get inside the tissue to do its work.

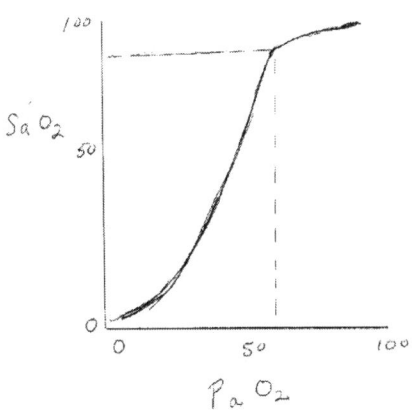

Hemoglobin Saturation Curve

There is even more to the hemoglobin molecule. It is a very large protein made up of chains of amino acids which are highly charged molecules. The carbon dioxide molecule is like water. It has a positive charged side and a negatively charged side:

$$\begin{array}{c} (-) \\ O \quad\quad O \\ C \\ (+) \end{array}$$

Thus, carbon dioxide can attach to the amino acids of hemoglobin using Van der Waals binding. When a CO_2 molecule attaches to hemoglobin it kicks off some of the oxygen. The same thing happens with the acid radical H^+. When H^+ attaches to hemoglobin by binding to the amine radical of an amino acid, it kicks off a molecule of oxygen from hemoglobin. These changes are called the *Bohr Effect* or the *shift to the right* of the hemoglobin saturation curve. The Bohr Effect also makes it easier to deliver oxygen to the tissues. Because of the active metabolism in the tissues, the levels of CO_2 and H^+ are high. Remember oxygen is consumed and carbon dioxide, and indirectly, hydrogen ion, are produced. We want oxygen to be unloaded at the tissue level. The opposite is true in the lungs where CO_2 and H^+ are low so the Hemoglobin Saturation curve shifts to the left making it easier to take up the oxygen.

There is a third compound, 2, 3 DPG, or *2, 3, diphosphoglycerate*, which is a product of metabolism, which also shifts the curve to the right. Finally, the temperature is higher at the tissue level where metabolism is actively going on. Higher temperatures also shift the curve to the right. Thus, in actively metabolizing tissue, the curve shifts to the right to help unload the Oxygen from hemoglobin.

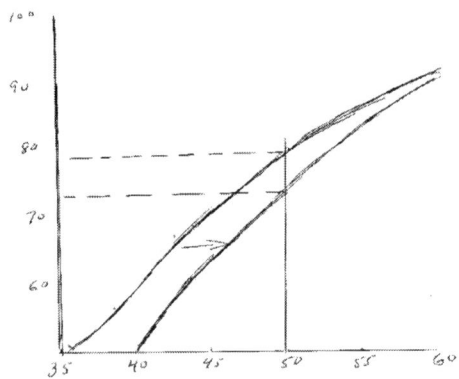

At a PaO_2 of 50 on the normal curve the SaO_2 is 78 but on the curve shifted to the right it is only 73. Oxygen is released with the "shift to the right".

The formula for the amount of oxygen per 100 cc of blood becomes:

Amount of dissolved O_2 in the blood + the amount of O_2 bound to hemoglobin

Or

$(.003 \times PaO_2) + (1.34 \times \text{Hemoglobin} \times SaO_2)$

Thus if a patient has a hemoglobin of 15, a PaO_2 of 60 and a SaO_2 of 90, the amount of oxygen will be:

$$(.003 \times 60) + (1.34 \times 15 \times .90)$$

Or

$$.18 + 18.1$$

Or

18.3 grams of Oxygen per 100 cc of blood

Carbon dioxide transport is, in some sense, much more complex. Carbon Dioxide can react with water to form carbonic acid:

$$CO_2 + H_2O > H_2CO_3$$

The carbonic acid can then break down into a hydrogen ion and a bicarbonate ion:

$$H_2CO_3 > H^+ + HCO_3^-$$

We can now ask how is CO_2 carried. The CO_2 can be dissolved in the blood or it can enter the red blood cell and attach to the hemoglobin, kicking off some oxygen, or while in the RBC, it can be combined with water to form H_2CO_3 which is metabolized to a hydrogen ion and a bicarbonate ion. The Hydrogen ion also binds to the hemoglobin, and the bicarbonate ion is then kicked out of the RBC in exchange for a chloride ion. This reaction is called *The Chloride Shift*.

All in all, 11% of the CO_2 is transported in plasma of which 1% is bound to protein, 5% is transported as the bicarbonate ion and 5% is dissolved in the blood. Thus, the majority of the CO_2 is transported in the red blood cell. In the RBC, about 21% is bound to hemoglobin, 5% is dissolved in the cytosol of the RBC, and 63% is carried as the bicarbonate ion.

Lastly, the difference between hypoxia and hypoxemia can be confusing:

Hypoxemia means low Oxygen in the blood

Hypoxia just means low Oxygen and it usually is applied to tissues.

What are the common causes of tissue hypoxia? We can classify hypoxia into four groups:

1. Hypoxemic
2. Anemic
3. Circulatory failure
4. Histotoxic

Hypoxemic hypoxia is tissue hypoxia due to low oxygen in the blood. The PaO_2 is low. This might be seen in a patient with asthma or heart failure.

With *Anemic hypoxia* the oxygen level as measured by the PaO_2 is normal but there is just not enough RBC's and hemoglobin to get an adequate amount of oxygen to the tissues. This can be seen in a patient who is bleeding profusely, or a patient with a severe anemia from a Vitamin B12 deficiency, or a patient who has an abnormal hemoglobin that doesn't work as well as hemoglobin A. Patients with Sickle Cell Anemia, an autosomal recessive genetic disorder, or patients who have methemoglobinemia, another genetic condition in which the iron molecule in the hemoglobin exists in the Fe^3 state instead of the Fe^2 state seen in normal hemoglobin, fit into this category.

In *Circulatory Hypoxia* the PaO_2 is normal and the hemoglobin is normal but the heart can't pump enough blood to satisfy the needs of the tissues for oxygen. This condition is most often due to congestive heart failure.

The last condition, *Histotoxic Hypoxia,* is certainly the most interesting. In this condition, the PaO_2 is normal, the hemoglobin is normal, and the circulation is normal. Still, the tissues are hypoxic. The hypoxia occurs because the mitochondria are shut down by a toxin. All the oxygen in the blood is just not going to be used by the inactive mitochondria. Thus sugar is broken down to pyruvate which is converted to lactic acid. This condition is seen with cyanide poisoning and in a patient with Septic Shock Syndrome. The blood gases in a patient with sepsis show a normal oxygen level but a marked acidosis with a decreased level of bicarbonate or HCO_3^- and increased lactic acid.

The White Blood Cells

The leucocytes or WBC's are the body's mobile defenders against foreign invaders. Some of the leucocytes (granulocytes and monocytes) phagocytose or destroy the invader; some of the leucocytes (some lymphocytes) produce antibodies which attach to the invader and make it easier for the phagocytes to destroy it.

Because the WBC's are blood-borne they are able to travel to any site in the body where infection or inflammation occurs, whether it is the lungs, the kidneys, the liver, or wherever. There are normally between 5,000 and 9,000 WBC's per milliliter.

There are five common types of leucocytes.

	TYPE	% of WBC's
1.	Lymphocytes:	30%
2.	Monocytes:	5.3%
3.	Neutrophil or PMN	62%
4.	Eosinophils	2.3%
5.	Basophils	0.4%

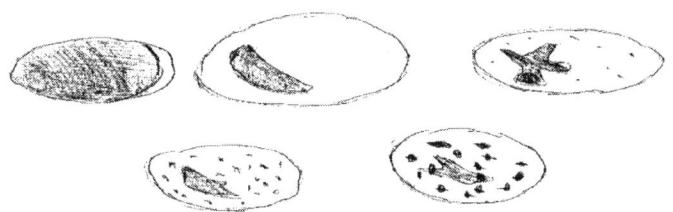

The figure at the top left is the <u>lymphocyte</u> which is a tiny cell made up mainly of its nucleus. The top middle figure is the *monocyte* which is much larger than the lymphocyte and has a lot more cytoplasm. The top right figure is the <u>neutrophil</u> which has a "lobed" nucleus and a few granules. In a serious infection there may be "band" neutrophils which are younger forms of the **PMN** or polymorphonuclear granulocyte. Instead of a lobed nucleus they have a single ribbon-like nucleus. The figure on the lower left is the <u>eosinophil</u> which has many bright red staining granules in its cytoplasm. The figure on the lower right is the <u>basophil</u> whose granules are large, dense, and stain dark blue.

The neutrophils, eosinophils and basophils all have granules in their cytoplasm and are referred to as "granulocytes". The eosinophilic granules stain deep red and the basophil granules stain dark blue on the Wright's Stain which is commonly used to color blood smears.

The granulocytes and monocytes are formed in the bone marrow while most of the lymphocytes, while formed in the bone marrow, must be activated by the thymus gland located in the upper anterior mediastinum, the lymph nodes scattered throughout our body or in patches of lymph tissue along our intestinal tract.

The granulocytes live only a few hours in the blood while the monocytes live much longer, up to 10 hours. The lymphocytes live for weeks or longer. The memory lymphocytes live even much longer than that.

When a patient gets pneumonia, the leucocytes are called to action. Cells in the lungs send signals called *chemotaxins* into the blood which attract the circulating leucocytes which travel from the blood to the site of the infection. They cross into the tissue by squeezing through the pores of the capillaries, a process called *diapedesis*. Even though the pores are tiny, much tinier than the WBC in fact, the cells are able to squirm their way through them. Once at the site of the invasion they crawl about like amoeba and attack the invaders.

When the monocyte reaches the infected tissue it changes into a macrophage, a very large phagocytic cell. Along with the neutrophils, the macrophages ingest and digest the invading bacteria or virus. They also have bactericidal chemicals which kill ingested bacteria.

After defeating the invader some of the macrophages will remain in the lung for months or years as *alveolar macrophages*.

The *eosinophils* are involved primarily in allergic reactions and to a lesser extent as a response to parasitic invaders. Parasites are too large for the eosinophils to ingest but the eosinophils have surface chemicals which allow them to attach in large number to the parasites and release substances which ultimately kill them.

The main role for the eosinophils is in the response to allergens, which are objects such as pollens which can cause an allergic reaction in some people. *Mast cells*, which are circulating basophils that have migrated into the tissue in response to an allergen, send out chemotaxins which attract the eosinophils. The mast cells of the lungs and nasal passages release vasoactive chemicals, such as histamines, which are responsible for the allergic symptoms. The eosinophils engulf and destroy the antigen-antibody complexes helping to ameliorate the allergic response. Allergic individuals have a high eosinophil count and are called *atopic*.

The basophils transform into *mast cells* when they are in tissues. When the antibody, IgE, attaches to the mast cell the mast cell ruptures releasing histamines (the chemicals which cause allergic symptoms), heparin (which thins the blood), as well as bradykinin, leukotrienes and serotonin, all of which can precipitate bronchospasm.

The lymphocyte is a fascinating but complex cell. There are two major groups of lymphocytes, the T lymphocytes and the B lymphocytes. They are called B and T because of where they originate in the chick embryo. The T cells originate in the Thymus gland and turn out to be important in *cellular immunity* while the B cells originate in the *Bursa of Fabricus* which are collections of lymphatic tissue in the gut of the embryo. These cells become the *Plasma Cells* which make antibodies and thus are important in *humeral immunity*.

There are several types of T lymphocytes. The two main groups are the T4 lymphocytes or *helper lymphocytes* and the T8 lymphocytes or *killer lymphocytes*. The T4 helper cells migrate to the site of a foreign invasion and attach themselves to the invader. Then they activate the B lymphocytes which become plasma cells and release antibodies against the invader. Without the T4 cells only tiny amounts of antibodies would be released. Some of the T4 lymphocytes then store the information about the invader and pass it on to their offspring so that whenever a similar invader returns, they will be able to respond immediately. Some of the B lymphocytes also form a memory of the invader. Thus, the body is always prepared. The T8 lymphocytes contain potent chemicals which destroy the invader.

The patient who suffers from the *Acquired Immunodeficiency Syndrome (AIDS)* has very low levels of T4 cells because the AIDS virus or *HIV (Human Immuno-Virus)* preferentially attaches to the CD4 receptors on the T4 cells. The virus then enters the cell and uses the cell's own metabolism to produce more viruses before destroying it. The death of the T4 cells makes the patient with AIDS very susceptible to common pathogens such as the pneumococcal bacterium.

Some of the T4 lymphocytes become *suppresser lymphocytes*. Once the invaders are destroyed the reaction must stop. After all, the neutrophils, macrophages, and lymphocytes are all releasing tons of chemicals such as proteinases and other enzymes into the tissue. If the reaction is not terminated, those proteinases will begin to destroy the tissues. They will become as bad as the invader. We will see how this happens when we discuss a type of emphysema known as *Alpha 1 Antitrypsin Deficiency*.

We will encounter T1 and T2 lymphocytes in our discussion of asthma and immunity.

Platelets

Platelets or *thrombocytes* are the tiny bits of cellular material that circulate in the blood looking for leaks in capillaries and large blood vessels to plug. They act like a glue to fasten the torn vessel together. There are normally about 300,000 platelets per milliliter.

They are even smaller than the RBC, 4 micra compared to 6-7 micra for the RBC. The platelets are born in the bone marrow from giant cells called megakaryocytes which fragment into hordes of cellular debris. They live in the blood for about 8 to 12 days.

While they don't have a nucleus, their cytoplasm has the contractile proteins actin and myosin, similar to the proteins that make up our muscles. They also have mitochondria which provide the ATP or Adenosine triphosphate for contracture to occur. They also have a type of growth hormone which encourages the lining of blood vessels to grow and repair.

Microvesicles

Microvesicles are very tiny (less than 1 micron) spheres filled with cytosol that originate from many different types of cells. They are packaged inside the cell, migrate to the surface and are extruded into the cell's environ. They contain protein, RNA and mitochondria. They function in cell communication. They have surface markers which can bind to cells. When the vesicle binds to the cell its contents can then be injected into the cell.

They have several functions. They are important in the immune function and inflammation. They are important in heart disease. Angiotensin 11 causes the release of microvesicles in the heart which causes hypertrophy of the cardiac muscle. Obesity causes the release of inflammatory vesicles. Likely they are very important in the development of cancer. They encourage the growth of cancer cells and may be the trigger for metastasis.

Peter A. Petroff, MD

IMPORTANT CONCEPTS TO REMEMBER FROM THIS LECTURE

1. What is the difference between the hemoglobin concentration and the hematocrit?

    The hemoglobin concentration is the grams of hemoglobin per 100 cc of blood. The hematocrit is the volume of the formed RBC elements divided by the total volume of a sample of blood.

2. What causes the shift to the right of the hemoglobin dissociation curve?

    The shift to the right is caused by products of metabolism at the tissue level including increased temperature, increased CO_2, increased 2,3 DPG, and decreased pH.

3. What is the difference between hypoxia and hypoxemia?

    Hypoxemia means low O_2 in the blood; hypoxia means low O_2 in the tissues.

4. Which type of white cell is associated with allergy

    The eosinophil

Lecture 3

The Heart: Anatomy and Physiology

The heart is a muscular structure the size of your clenched fist located in the anterior part of your chest directly behind the sternum. It sits on top of the diaphragm and is bounded on both sides by the lungs.

The heart has four chambers, two atria and two ventricles, as well as four valves: the tricuspid, pulmonary, mitral and aortic. It is innervated by the sympathetic and parasympathetic nervous systems which act on the "pacemakers" of the heart. The "neural" pathways inside the heart are actually specialized muscle cells which make the heart unique.

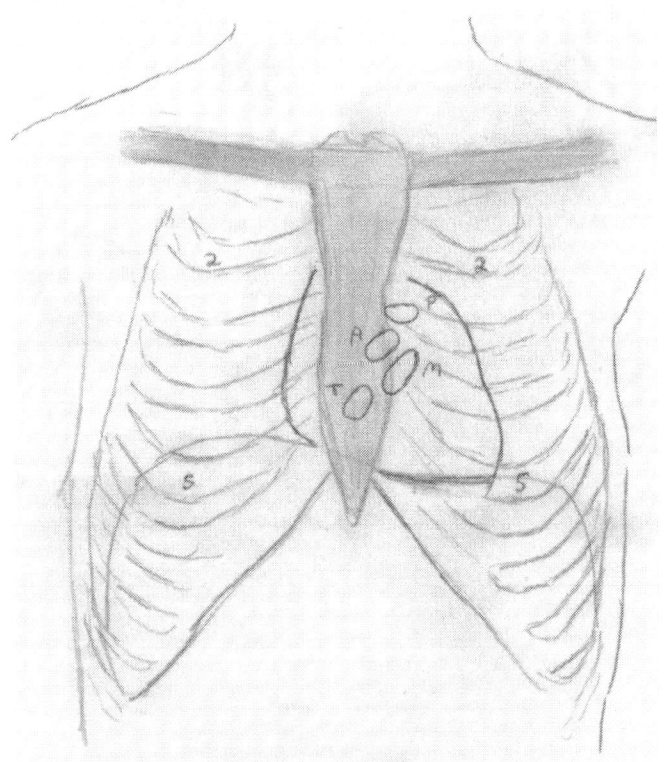

Heart in relation to the Chest Wall

The heart lies directly behind the sternum. The apex of the heart is located at the 5th rib in the mid-clavicular line (draw a line from the middle of the clavicle downwards to where it intersects the fifth rib. The aortic sound is best heard in the 2nd rib interspace to the right of the sternum. The pulmonic sounds are best heard in the 2nd rib interspace to the left of the sternum. The positions of the valves are also indicated on the drawing. *A* is aortic valve, *P* is pulmonic valve, *M* is the mitral valve, and *T* is the tricuspid valve.

It is important to understand where the heart and valves are located with respect to surface markers. The apex of the heart, which is the left ventricle, is just outside the left edge of the sternum at the mid clavicular line at about the 5th rib interspace. The rest of the heart lies behind the sternum. When you touch the area of the apex you can feel the heart beating. The impulse that you feel is normally less than the size of a quarter. If it is much larger than a quarter the heart may be enlarged. The mitral valve directs blood flow from the left atrium into the left ventricle so the best place to hear mitral sounds is at the apex of the heart.

Blood flows from the left ventricle through the aortic valve towards the right shoulder. Therefore the best place to hear sounds generated by the aortic valve is in the 2nd right interspace next to the sternum.

Blood flows from the right ventricle upwards and slightly to the left into the main pulmonary artery through the pulmonary valve. Because of this, the best place to hear pulmonary valvular sounds is at the 2nd left intercostal space adjacent to the sternum. Pulmonary sounds are especially important to listen to in infants. The pulmonary valve is sometimes narrowed, a condition called pulmonary stenosis, and the murmur of pulmonary stenosis is best heard in the 2nd left interspace.

Mediastinum

The heart lies inside an envelope-like structure called the *pericardium*. The heart and its sac lie in the *mediastinum*. The mediastinum is the space in the center of the chest, like the core of an apple. It is bounded on the back by the spine (vertebral column), on the front by the sternum, and on the sides by the outer lining of the sac that encases the lungs, called the parietal pleural.

The mediastinum is packed with important structures. We can divide it into three parts, a superior part located above the heart which contains the trachea, thymus, and esophagus as well as some blood vessels and nerves, an anterior inferior part which is basically filled by the heart alongside of which run the phrenic nerves, and a posterior inferior part in which we find the esophagus, the aorta and the inferior vena cava.

Almost directly above the heart in the superior mediastinum is the carina of the trachea. This is the point where the trachea divides into the right and left main bronchial tubes. The trachea descends from the neck and divides into the right and left main stem bronchi just above the heart. The right main stem bronchus passes alongside the right atrium, which is covered by the pericardium. Thus, lung cancers involving the right main stem bronchus can invade the pericardium and cause inflammation in the pericardial sac and serious cardiac arrhythmias. Both major bronchi pass into the hila or "roots" of the lungs.

The tiny Thymus Gland is located directly in front of the trachea. It is usually atrophied in adults. However, on occasions, the Thymus can grow and become a tumor called a Thymoma. This is often seen in patients with a neurologic condition called Myasthenia Gravis which we will discuss in a later lecture.

The Superior Vena Cava vein is located to the right of the trachea. Cancers that involve the right side of the trachea can block the Superior Vena Cava causing swelling and cyanosis of the head and right arm. The Inferior Vena Cava enters the chest through a hole in the diaphragm, ascends and merges with the Superior Vena Cava, as they enter the right atrium.

The esophagus is located directly in back of the trachea in the superior mediastinum. After the trachea divides, the esophagus descends behind the heart and continues downwards, finally passing through a hole in the diaphragm into the abdomen to enter the stomach.

The aorta arises from the top of the left ventricle. At first it courses towards the right shoulder, then arches towards the left and back, across the top of the heart, to make a giant bend, called the "aortic arch". Then it descends behind the heart through the diaphragm into the abdomen. Shortly after crossing the diaphragm it will give off branches to the kidneys, called the Renal Arteries, as well as the gut, called the Superior and Inferior Mesenteric Arteries, and finally divide into the Iliac Arteries which supply our pelvis and legs with blood.

The Pulmonary Artery arises from the top of the right ventricle, just behind and to the right of the Aorta. It ascends with a slight leftward tilt then abruptly divides into the right and left pulmonary arteries which enter the hila of the lungs.

The Mediastinum is also filled with nerves including the sympathetic and parasympathetic nerves which innervate the heart and lungs as well as the Phrenic Nerves which innervates the diaphragm. There are lymph channels and copious lymph nodes. Blood vessels in the Superior Mediastinum include the Internal Carotids, which provide blood to our brains, and the Subclavian Arteries, which provide nourishment to our arms.

The Structure of the Heart

The heart is a large mass of muscle. It is divided into four chambers: two atria and two ventricles. It is also divided into a right side and a left side. Thus there is a right atrium, right ventricle, left atrium and left ventricle.

The right side of the heart is the "low-pressure" side of the heart. The left side of the heart is the "high-pressure" side of the heart. The right side of the heart supplies blood to the lungs. The left side of the heart supplies blood to all the major organs of the body, from the brain all the way down to the tip of the toes. Thus, the walls of the left atrium and especially the left ventricle must have much more muscle and be much thicker than the walls of the right atrium and right ventricle.

The heart sits in a sac called the pericardium. The pericardium has two layers, an outer, more fibrous layer called the *Parietal Pericardium* and a thin, inner layer, which also forms the outermost layer of the heart itself, called the *Visceral Pericardium*. Between the Parietal and the Visceral Pericardium is a virtual space. The pericardial space can sometimes become filled with fluid, or even blood, which causes the heart to fail by not allowing it to relax fully and fill with blood during diastole. If the heart can't fill with blood during diastole, it can't deliver enough blood to the organs that depend on it. This condition, called pericardial tamponade, occurs with viral infections, tuberculosis, and with cancers, especially lung cancers.

The wall of the heart consists of three layers: 1. the outermost layer which is one cell layer thick is actually the visceral pericardium, 2. the thick mass of muscle, and 3. the inner layer lining the heart. The outermost layer is called the *Epicardium;* the muscle mass is called the *Myocardium* and the innermost layer is called the *Endocardium*. The epicardium and endocardium are made up of *Squamous Cells* similar to the cells of our skin. The pericardium is only one layer thick but the endocardium is much thicker. The endocardium is contiguous with the lining of the blood vessels entering and leaving the heart. It also covers all the valves of the heart.

The blood vessels that supply the heart lie on the surface of the epicardium and send branches deep into the muscle mass of the heart.

The heart has four valves: tricuspid, pulmonary, mitral and aortic.

The valves are important in that they permit the blood to travel in only one direction. For example, the mitral valve lies between the left atrium and the left ventricle. When the left atrium contracts, it will force blood past the open Mitral Valve into the left ventricle but when the left ventricle contracts, the Mitral Valve will be shut tight and the blood can't go back into the left atrium. This is true for all the valves.

Two problems can go wrong with the valves. They can either become too narrow, which is called *stenosis,* or they can become leaky, which is called *regurgitation.* The most common valvular disorder in adults is Mitral Regurgitation in which the Mitral Valve is *incompetent* or leaky and allows blood to flow backwards from the left ventricle into the left atrium. This is often seen in Congestive Heart Failure. The second most common valvular disorder in adults is Aortic Stenosis. The Aortic Valve becomes stiff and is unable to open enough for blood to exit the left ventricle into the aorta during systole. This condition is often seen with aging or in patients who were born with two aortic cusps instead of the normal three cusps.

Posterior

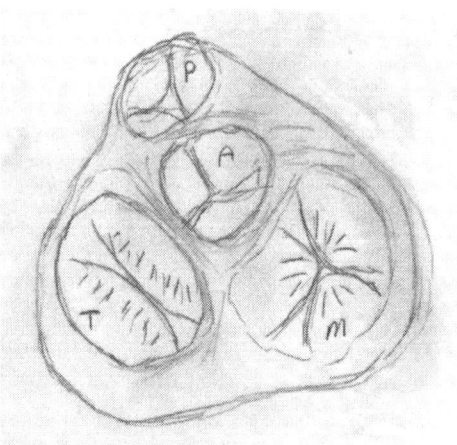

Anterior

This is a view of the heart with the atria removed. It is evident that the valves are contiguous. The Tricuspid Valve (T) has two leaflets and is located anteriorly and on the right. Opposite it is the Mitral Valve (M), which has three leaflets. The Aortic Valve (A) lies directly behind and a little between the Tricuspid and Aortic Valves. The Pulmonic Valve (P) lies at the right posterior margin of the heart. Both the Aortic Valve and the Pulmonic Valve have three leaflets or cusps.

The heart is innervated by both the Sympathetic Nervous System and the Parasympathetic Nervous System. Both supply nerves to the Sinoatrial Node (SA node), which is the primary pacemaker of the heart and the Atrioventricular Node (AV node) which is the secondary pacemaker. The Sympathetic Nervous System secretes Adrenaline which causes the heart to beat faster and stronger. The Parasympathetic Nervous System secretes Acetyl Choline, which slows the heart.

The blood supply to the heart comes from the coronary arteries. The coronary arteries arise from the Aorta just after it emerges from the heart. The Left Coronary Artery provides the main supply of blood to the enormous left ventricle. It divides into a Circumflex Artery which wraps around the heart to a portion of the backside of the heart and the Anterior Descending Artery which supplies blood to the entire left ventricle. Most of the posterior and inferior wall of the heart is supplied by the much smaller Right Coronary Artery. If a blockage occurs to the Anterior Descending Artery, the entire left ventricle will die. That is why a blockage in the Anterior Descending Artery is called the "widow maker".

The coronary arteries fill only during *diastole* when the heart muscle is relaxed. In addition, the time allowed for the heart to contract (*systole*) is a constant. It doesn't change no matter how fast the heart beats. The heart can only contract so fast. The time for contraction is the same at a heart rate of 70 as it is at a heart rate of 140. Therefore, the time the heart spends in diastole must shorten the faster the heart beats. Thus, with a very fast heart rate there will be little time for the coronary arteries to fill and supply blood effectively to the heart.

Circulation of the blood in the heart

The circulation of the blood in the heart is fairly straight-forward. Blood flows from the vena cava into the right atrium, then through the tricuspid valve into the right ventricle. The right side of the heart is the low pressure side of the heart. The peak pressures in the right ventricle are normally about 12 to 18 mm Hg. When the right ventricle contracts, the tricuspid valve slams shut. The blood flows from the right ventricle, across the pulmonic valve into the pulmonary artery. It is called an artery because it flows away from the heart. *Arteries flow away from the heart; veins flow towards the heart.* The pulmonic valve closes as the right ventricle begins to relax. As it relaxes, the pressure in the right ventricle becomes less than the pressure in the pulmonary artery forcing the pulmonic valve to close. The pulmonary artery divides again and again till finally it becomes the small capillaries of the lung which surround the alveoli, then the capillaries merge and merge again and again, ultimately forming the pulmonary vein which empties into the left atrium.

Blood flows from the left atrium, across the mitral valve into the left ventricle. This is the high pressure side of the heart with peak pressures of 120 to 140 mm Hg in the left ventricle. When the left ventricle contracts during systole, the pressure in the left ventricle becomes much higher than the pressure in the left atrium and the mitral valve closes. Finally, the blood leaves the left ventricle across the aortic valve into the aorta. With left ventricular contraction, the pressure rises abruptly in the left ventricle forcing the aortic valve to open. Then, when the left ventricle begins to relax in diastole, the pressure in the aorta becomes much greater than the pressure in the left ventricle and the valve closes.

The Heart's Electrical System

The heart has two types of muscle. One type is strictly for contraction. One type is strictly for conducting electrical signals through the heart in order to coordinate the heart's action. In order to understand how the heart's electrical system works we need to understand the *Action Potential*.

The cell wall is made up of lipids which are hydrophobic. Water and charged ions can't get in and out of the cell easily. Instead there are channels, made up of large glycoprotein molecules which can open and close. If the cell wall were freely permeable, the concentration of sodium and potassium would be equal in the cell and in the extracellular space. Instead, the concentration of sodium outside the cell is about 144 meq/l while it is only about 7 meq/l inside the cell, a twenty-fold difference! The reverse is true for potassium. Inside the cell the potassium concentration is 144 meq/l and outside the cell it is about 4.4 meq/l. The difference between inside and outside concentration is maintained by the sodium and potassium channels. In muscle cells, there is also a channel for Calcium. The calcium level inside the cell is about 1 meq/l while outside the cell it is about 5 meq/l.

Because the potassium channel is a little leaky and the gradient between the inside and outside potassium level is so enormous, the potassium ion tends to diffuse out of the cell. When it does, it takes its positive charge with it, leaving behind a negatively charged ion such as chloride. Eventually the difference in electrical charge between the inside and outside of the cell puts a halt to the potassium's exodus from the cell but the outside of the muscle cell is now relatively positively charged compared to the inside of the cell. Thus there is a balance between electrical charge and diffusion. The inside of the cell is normally about – 90 mv with respect to the outside of the cell.

When the heart muscle cell is stimulated, the sodium channel opens. Because of the sheer number of positively charged sodium ions outside the cell compared to the inside, the sodium ions flood into the cell and the cell rapidly becomes positively charged. This influx of sodium deforms the cell. The deformation of the cell activates the muscle cells nearby to it and the "current" flows throughout the heart. The activation of the cell is referred to as the *Action Potential*.

In skeletal muscle, there is only a fast sodium channel, which when activated floods the interior of the muscles cells with sodium and causes the muscle to contract. In heart muscle there is also a slow sodium-calcium channel which opens when the sodium channel closes and which causes a much more prolonged contraction.

After the cell has been activated and begins to contract, the sodium and calcium channel close, the positively charged potassium is allowed to flow out of the cell through the potassium channel which returns the cell to its normal electrical (or "charged") state. Then the sodium and potassium pumps become activated. Sodium is kicked out of the cell and potassium drawn back into.

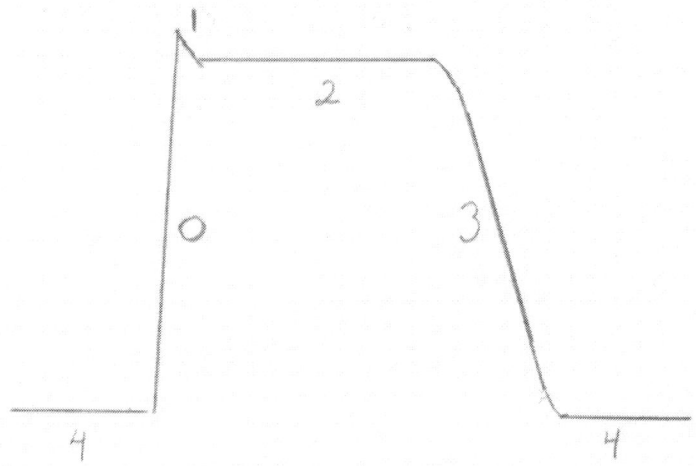

The Action Potential

The heart muscle is at rest in phase four, at about -90 mv. With excitation the cell rapidly *depolarizes* (phase zero) as the positively charged sodium ions flow into the cell. The charge inside the cell actually becomes positive, up to about + 70 mv. At phase one the potassium flows out of the cell partially repolarizing the cell. In phase two the calcium channel opens and the calcium flows into the cell balancing the exodus of the potassium ions, allowing the cell to maintain a charged state and a prolonged depolarization. In phase three, the calcium channel closes but potassium channel is still open allowing the potassium to flow out of the cell bringing the charge inside the cell back to baseline (phase four). Over time, the sodium, potassium, and calcium channels return the cell to its baseline state.

The difference between a normal muscle cell and a heart muscle cell is the calcium channel. The influx of calcium allows the cell to maintain its contraction longer. When we walk we don't want to do a "moon-walk". We really want to move. But in the heart we want the muscle to slowly squeeze out all the blood that it can. A fast contraction will raise the pressures inside the aorta catastrophically high and we might blow a fuse as those pressures are transmitted to our brain. No, slow and steady wins the race.

The depolarization of the heart muscle cell activates a calcium channel on the muscle cell's endoplasmic reticulum, or "cell highway", which in this case is called the *sarcoplasmic reticulum* instead of the *endoplasmic reticulum* as in other cells. The calcium leaks out of the sarcoplasmic reticulum into the cytosol of the cell and binds to Troponin, a large protein, which is located on the Actin molecules. The Actin forms cross-bridges with Myosin and the heart muscle contracts. The Calcium is then pumped back into the sarcoplasmic reticulum and out of the cell and the heart muscle relaxes.

When heart muscle is damaged such as during a heart attack, Troponin leaks out of the cell and can be measured in the blood.

The difference between muscle cells in the heart that simply squeeze out blood and the muscle cells that are pacemakers is in phase four of the action potential. The pacemaker cells have leaky sodium channels. The sodium slowly leaks into the cell. The charge inside the cells drops from minus 70 or so to minus 40; when that occurs the action potential fires.

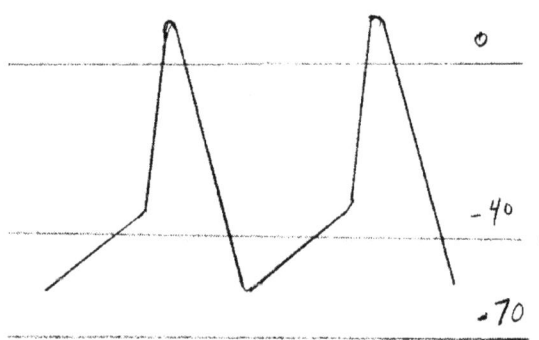

Pacemaker Action Potential

Instead of a flat phase four, there is a continuous sodium channel leak resulting in a progressive depolarization of the cell even when the cell is at rest. When the cell loses about half of its negativity it fires off its action potential. However, the calcium channel is not opened so the action potential resembles that of a nerve, rather than a heart muscle.

Each of the pacemaker cells has its own rate of sodium channel leakage. Thus the main pacemaker of the heart located in the sinoatrial node has the fastest leak and the cells fire about seventy times a minute whereas the pacemaker type cells in the ventricles have a much slower intrinsic sodium leakage so they only fire about fifteen to forty times a minute on their own. Because of that difference, the cells in the sinoatrial node are the primary pacemaker cells of the heart. They overwhelm the ventricular pacemaker cells.

In order to prevent a runaway rhythm, the heart muscles become unresponsive or only partially responsive to electrical signals during parts of their action potential. The *absolute refractory period* is the time when nothing will stimulate the heart muscle cells to fire. This occurs in phases zero, one, two, and the first part of the third phase of the action potential. In the last part of phase three, the cell has a *relative refractory period* when a strong stimulus might trigger the heart muscle cell to fire again.

The Conducting System

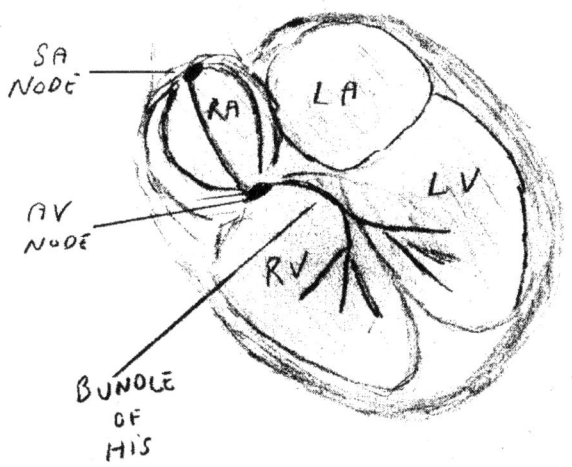

The Conduction System of the Heart.

The primary pacemaker of the heart is the *sinoatrial node* (SA node) which is located in the right atrium near where the superior vena cava enters the heart. It consists of about 10,000 cells. Three *internodal channels* lead from the SA node to the *atrioventricular node* (AV node) which is located near the junction of the atria and ventricles, in the right atrium behind the tricuspid valve. The AV nodal cells have an intrinsic rate of about 60, much slower than the SA node, so the SA node is in charge. The AV node also acts as a delay between the SA node and the Purkinje fibers, which gives time for the atria to contract and fill the ventricles. The *Bundle of His* (also called the *atrioventricular bundle*) is made up of large Purkinje fibers which carry the signal into the ventricles where tit branches into a left and right bundle. *The Bundle of His allows only one-way conduction.* Signals from the ventricle cannot flow back into the atria. The conduction through the AV node is slow, but the conduction through the bundle and its branches, the Purkinje fibers, is very fast. The ventricles are rapidly depolarized which causes an organized synchronous contraction of the ventricles.

The sympathetic and parasympathetic nervous systems act directly on the SA node. The sympathetic system increases the rate of firing by releasing adrenaline, a Beta adrenergic agent. Maximum stimulation can triple the rate of firing and double the strength of contraction of the heart. The parasympathetic slows the rate of firing by releasing acetylcholine. Moderate stimulation of the parasympathetic system can cut the rate of firing in half. Strong stimulation can stop the SA node and slow conduction through the AV node resulting in syncope.

IMPORTANT CONCEPTS TO REMEMBER FROM THIS LECTURE

1. Rapid depolarization is due to?

    – The rapid influx of sodium into the cell along its pressure gradient.

2. A pacemaker cell is characterized by?

    – A slow leak of sodium into the cell which triggers an action potential at about -40 mV, and a slow return to baseline in order to prevent the pacemaker from re-exciting too soon.

3. How much does systole shorten when the heart beats faster?

    – Systole does not shorten; diastole shortens.

4. Where is the thymus located?

    – Directly in front of the trachea in the superior mediastinum

Lecture Four
The EKG or Electrocardiogram

The Normal EKG

The first and most important concept about the EKG is that it does NOT measure how well the heart contracts. In fact, it has NOTHING to do with contraction of the heart. It only measures the ELECTRICAL ACTIVITY of the heart. You can have a normal EKG but have absolutely NO cardiac output. The EKG can look great, but the heart can be as dead as a cell-phone whose battery has run out of charge!

As the heart depolarizes, its surface changes from positive to negative as the positive sodium ions move from outside to the inside of the cell. A tiny electrical current is formed. This electrical current can be measured even on the surface of the body. It is a very small current measured in microvolts, but it is still measurable.

The electrical signal of the heart goes from the SA node near the top and to the right of the sternum to the left ventricle at the bottom of the heart to the left of the sternum. Basically it follows a path similar to the line drawn from the right shoulder down to the left foot.

If we put very sensitive electrodes on the right shoulder, left shoulder, and left foot, we will

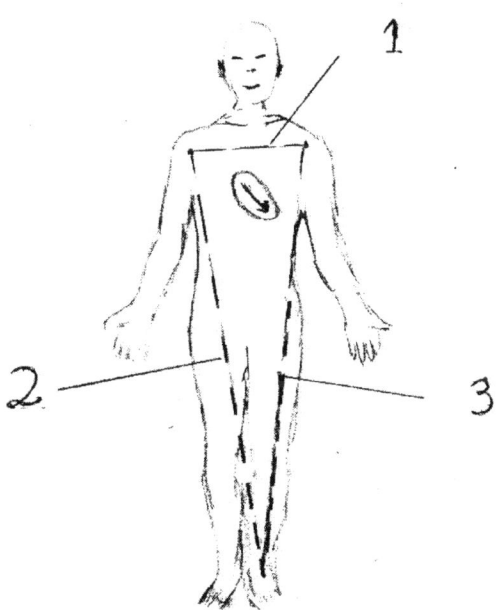

Leads 1, 2, 3, related to the electrical signal of the heart

find that the signal from the right shoulder to the left foot (2) is parallel to the signal traversing the heart, as is the line from the right shoulder to the left shoulder (1) while lead 3 from the left foot to the left shoulder goes in an opposite direction. In fact lead 2, the lead from the right shoulder to the left foot, is the best approximation to the direction of the electrical system in the heart. This is the lead you will see most often on the monitors in the Intensive Care Unit. In some individuals, especially the very overweight patient, lead 1 may work better.

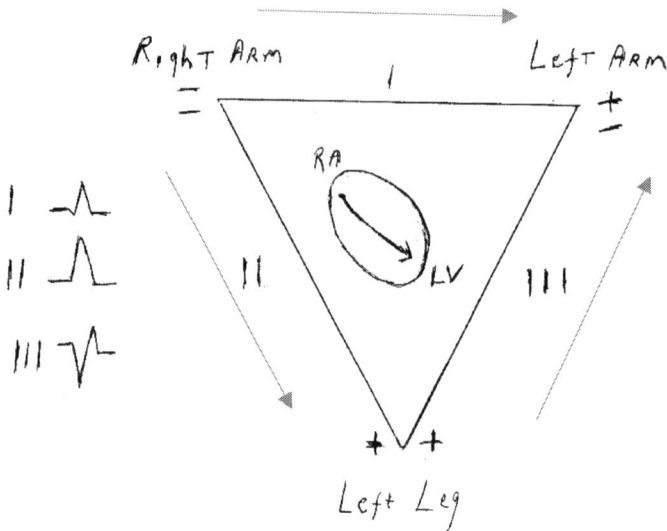

The schematic shows the relationship between the heart and the three main leads. Leads 1 and 2 are always parallel to the heart and provide the best signal to look at cardiac arrhythmias.

There are several other leads on an EKG including the unipolar leads and the frontal leads. These leads are more important for diagnosing heart damage and not arrhythmias.

The EKG tracing consists of lots of tiny squares. The X axis goes left to right and represents time. The Y axis goes up and down and represents voltage. Each little square going up and down is 0.1 millivolt. Each little square on the X axis represents 0.04 seconds. Thus each big line on the X axis is 0.2 seconds and five big lines is 1 second.

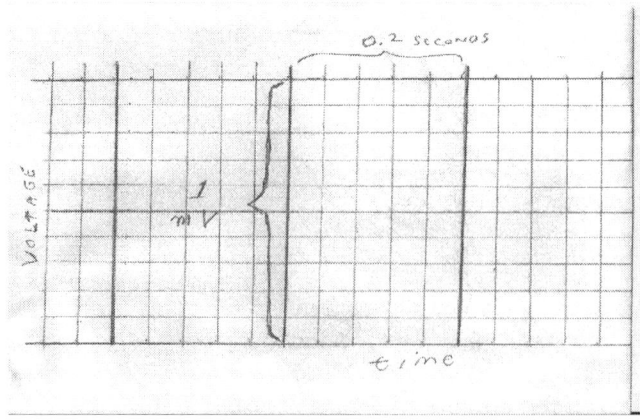

Each big line on the time line is 0.2 seconds; each small line is 0.04 seconds

The normal EKG pattern includes a small upward deflection at the onset of depolarization of the heart. This is called the P wave and represents atrial depolarization. The line returns to baseline and there is then a pause before the next big deflection occurs, which represents ventricular depolarization. This is called the QRS complex because, most often, the complex begins with a slight downward deflection (Q), then a large upright deflection (R) and then another downward deflection (S) before the line returns to baseline. The QRS complex is due to ventricular **depolarization** and because the ventricles have much more muscle mass than the atria it is much larger than the P wave. There is another pause and then a last upward deflection called the T wave which represents ventricular **repolarization**. Occasionally some patients will have still another upward deflection. This is called the U wave and is most often seen in patients with low potassium (hypokalemia).

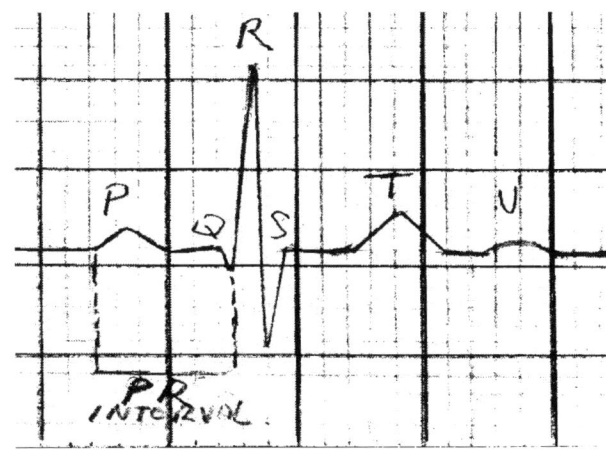

Normal EKG pattern

The P wave is normally about 0.08 to .11 seconds long. It is a smooth upright deflection with an amplitude of less than 2 mV (two small squares), but in patients with cor pulmonale it is often peaked and shaped like a tent, with a height of more than 2.5 millivolts (2 and a half little lines up).

The time between the onset of the P wave and the onset of the QRS is called the PR interval. The PR interval represents the delay in the AV node which allows for the time needed for atrial contraction. The PR interval is between .12 and .20 seconds.

The QRS complex measures from 0.08 to 0.12 seconds and represents ventricular depolarization. Normally the Q is very small. The R wave is the largest deflection. The time between the onset of the Q wave and the end of the T wave is called the QT interval and is about 0.36 seconds. The T wave represents ventricular repolarization. At the end of the T wave the heart has returned to baseline electrically.

A normal EKG has a P wave for every QRS and a QRS for every P wave. In addition the time for electrical excitation is within the normal limits.

We can measure the ventricular rate easily if the rhythm is regular by taking the number of large squares between two successive R waves and dividing that number into three hundred. For example if the R waves are exactly three large squares apart, the heart rate is 300/3 or 100. If the distance between two R waves is 3.6 big squares (three big squares and three little squares) the heart rate is 300/3.6 or 83. If the rhythm is irregular than count the number of R waves in three seconds (15 large squares) and multiple by 20.

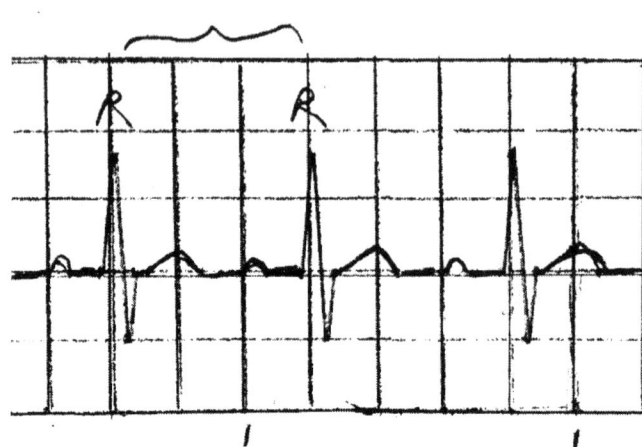

The two R waves are exactly three large squares apart.

Divide 300 by 3 to get a heart rate of 100.

Cardiac arrhythmias

Cardiac arrhythmias can be divided into several large groups.

1. Sinus Arrhythmias
2. Atrial Arrhythmias
3. Ventricular arrhythmias
4. Heart Blocks
5. Artificial Pacemaker Rhythms

Sinus dysrhythmias

Sinus rhythm is characterized simply by the expression: "Every P has a QRS". If you see a P wave for every QRS, the patient is in sinus rhythm and his EKG looks like the one drawn on the prior page and above. The normal heart rate is between 60 and 100. If the sinus rhythm is less than 60, the patient has *Sinus Bradycardia*. If the heart rate is greater than 100, the patient has *Sinus Tachycardia*.

Sinus bradycardia can be a sign of disease, such as *heroin overdose* or *hypothyroidism* (too little thyroid hormone), or it can be seen in patients taking a type of medication called a Beta Blocker. But it can even be found in people who exercise a lot and who are in extremely good health such as marathoners.

Sinus tachycardia can occur with stress such as taking one of the exams of this course, or with diseases such as *hyperthyroidism,* in which the thyroid gland produces too much thyroid hormone, *anemia, hypoxia, congestive heart failure, fever, exercise* or *shock*. It can also be seen in patients who are taking B *adrenergic agents* such as *albuterol,* or who take a cold preparation that contains *ephedrine,* or even after a large cup of coffee or glass of tea.

There is one other very interesting sinus dysrhythmia called *Sinus Arrhythmia.* in which the heart rate varies with inspiration and expiration. The heart rate is faster in inspiration and slower in expiration. The heart rate changes because of reflex changes in vagal tone during the different stages of the respiratory cycle. Inspiration increases the heart rate by decreasing vagal tone. The opposite happens in exhalation. This is often seen in children and young adults and is totally normal.

Atrial Arrhythmias

Atrial Arrhythmias are characterized by absent or deformed P waves associated with totally normal QRS complexes. For some reason the patient's SA node is no longer acting as the pacemaker. The SA node has been replaced by another pacemaker in the atria. However the QRS complex is normal because conduction through the AV node is preserved and the ventricles fire normally. In this case, the AV nodes also block some of the signals. The atria on their own can fire up to 360 times a minute, but the ventricles can contract, at most, two hundred or so times a minute. If the ventricular rate goes any faster, the coronary arteries can't supply enough blood to the heart. Thus, the AV node acts as a regulator to preserve the heart function.

The simplest atrial arrhythmia is the *premature atrial contraction (PAC)*. Most adults have an occasional PAC. If you drink a lot of coffee or tea you may have a lot of PAC's. A PAC is due to a tiny focus in the atria escaping from the control of the SA node and firing on its own. For some reason it has become a little twitchy. The PAC can be differentiated from the more serious *premature ventricular contraction (PVC)* because the PAC does not reset the heart rhythm. Thus when you listen you hear a regular rhythm which suddenly is interrupted by an unexpected beat but then goes on as if nothing had happened. In contrast, the PVC resets the rhythm so that, after a PCV, the rhythm begins anew with the PVC.

With a PAC, the P wave may or may not be seen. If it is seen it will be different from the normal P wave. It may be inverted, bi-lobed (shaped like an Asian camel's double hump), or just smaller. Sometimes, it may even come after the QRS or be buried in the QRS complex. If the P wave appears before the QRS, the PR interval will be shorter than normal. The QRS or ventricular complex will be normal in shape as will the QT interval. Normally there is a compensatory pause after the PAC but it is not as long as the compensatory pause after a premature ventricular contraction.

The treatment of PAC's is more often than not worse than the disease itself. If the patient has a heart or lung condition causing frequent PAC's treat the heart or lung condition not the PAC's.

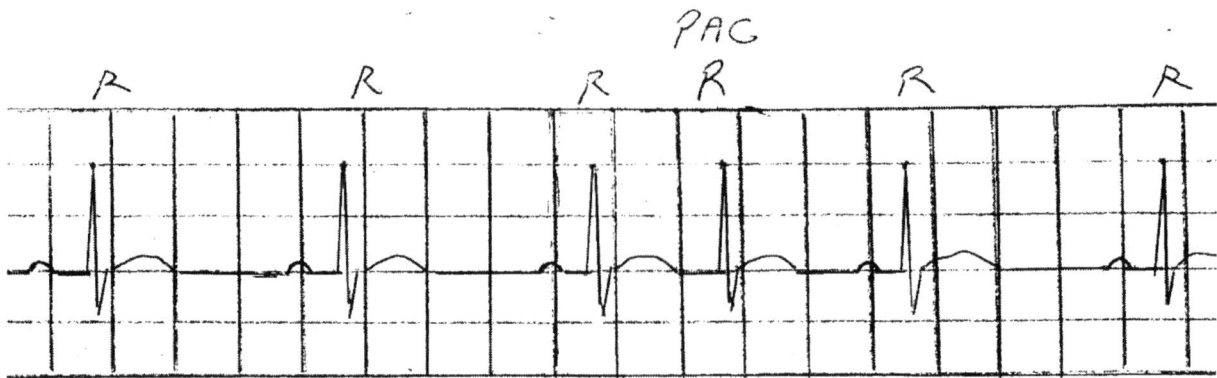

There is a single PAC occurring after the second QRS Complex. It occurs after two large squares rather than four. The PAC shows a normal QRS complex and T waves. There is compensatory pause which is far shorter than two P-P intervals.

A more serious condition is <u>*paroxysmal atrial tachycardia (PAT)*</u>. This arrhythmia may occur spontaneously or run in families in a condition called the Wolff Parkinson White Syndrome.

PAT is characterized clinically by the sudden onset of a rapid pulse which, depending upon the patient's age, may be asymptomatic or have serious symptoms such as shortness of breath, chest pain, or even fainting (syncope). The tachycardia then ends just as suddenly as it began. The electrocardiogram is diagnostic of the disorder. The rhythm of PAT is totally regular but there are no normal P waves to be seen. Still the QRS complexes and the T waves are totally normal. It is as if the P waves have just vanished. Occasionally with very close observation the missing P waves can be seen hidden in the QRS complex but this is an unusual finding.

PAT is due to the electrical signal arising from a point in the atria and creating a loop along an accessory pathway. The atria fire at a rate of 300 but the AV node blocks the signal so that the heart rate is usually exactly 150 (a 2:1 block).

PAT can be seen in patients with heart or lung disease but is most often seen as a hereditary syndrome called *Wolff Parkinson White Syndrome* in which there is an auxiliary atrial pathway. Prolonged PAT can cause the heart to weaken and sometimes can degenerate into more serious arrhythmias so it should be treated aggressively. Spontaneous PAT is treated with medicines such as *Adenosine,* whereas WPW is treated by identifying and destroying the auxiliary pathways.

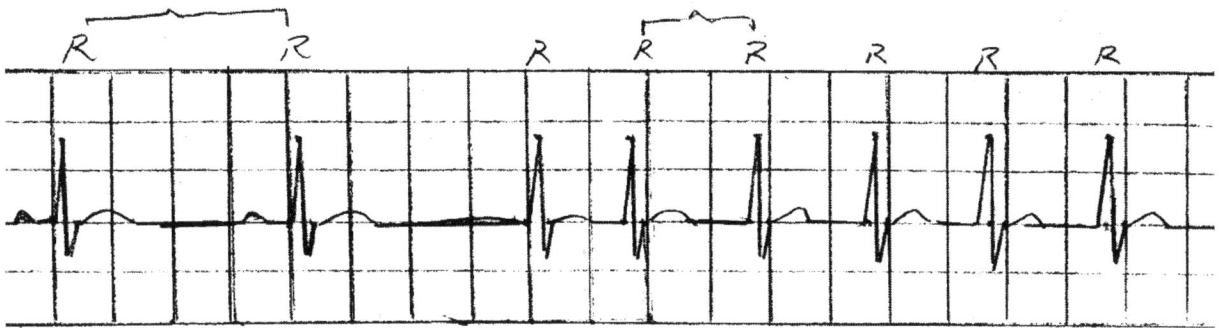

The onset of the PAT occurs with the third QRS complex. Suddenly, the P waves are gone and the QRS complexes now are occurring every second large square for a rate of 300/2 or 150. But the QRS complexes are totally normal.

Atrial Flutter is a more serious atrial arrhythmia which usually indicates the presence of significant underlying heart disease. Clinically it occurs in older individuals and, again, it may or may not be symptomatic, depending upon how fast the ventricular contractions occur. If the pulse is below a hundred the patient will likely not even know that he has atrial flutter. If the pulse is 150 and the patient is older or has blockage in his coronary arteries, he or she will be short of breath and often have angina.

The diagnosis of atrial flutter is easily established using the EKG. Classically *saw tooth waves* are seen instead of P waves. The saw tooth waves represent the circular electrical current in the atria. Instead of an electrical signal running from the SA node to the AV node along three fast pathways, the electrical signal is beginning somewhere in the atria and then running down to the AV node then back into the atria in a vicious cycle. Again the AV node blocks some of the signals. Most often there is a 2:1 block and the heart rate is 150, but the block can even be 4:1 and the heart rate will be only 75. The QRS complexes are totally normal. Conduction from the AV node to the ventricles is just as it should be.

Treatment is to electrically convert the signal back to normal though sometimes carotid massage is tried first. Carotid massage will slow the heart rate and allow the patient to convert to sinus rhythm spontaneously. There is a baroreceptor in the carotid body which when stimulated will send a signal along the parasympathetic nervous system to the lower part of the brain and then back to the AV node to increase the block and stop the atrial flutter.

Since the carotids provide the brain with oxygen, blocking both carotids for one or two minutes while you watch the EKG will not have a good outcome.

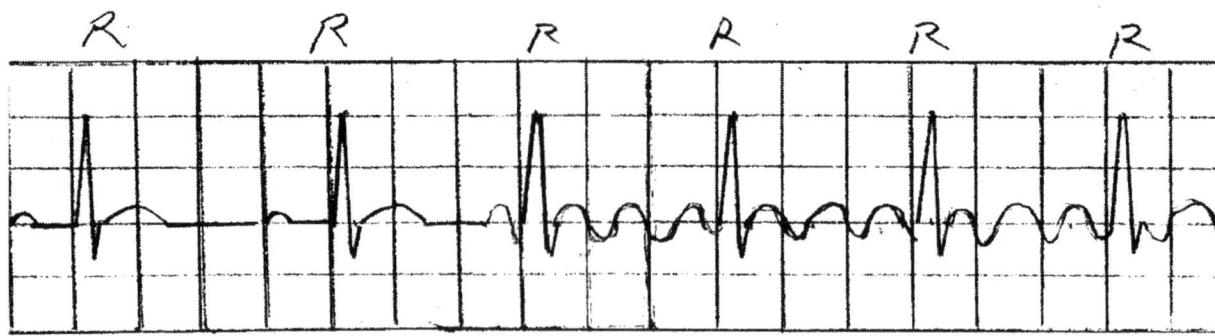

In this rhythm strip, Atrial Flutter begins suddenly on the third beat. The rhythm is still regular at a rate of 100 since the R to R distance is 3 (300/3 = 100). The QRS complexes are normal. The P waves have been replaced by a saw tooth wave.

The last atrial arrhythmia and the most important from our standpoint is *atrial fibrillation*. This heart rhythm can easily be diagnosed at the bedside. The rhythm is irregularly irregular. In other words a patient who has a lot of PAC's could have a rhythm that has a quick beat every third beat:

         1   2 3   1   2 3   1   2 3

This rhythm is irregular, because the third beat always occurs early. But it is danceable. It is *regularly irregular*. It's like a tango.

But the patient with atrial fibrillations has a rhythm where, no matter how you try, you just can't dance to it. It is totally irregular.

         1   2 3 4 5 6 7 8   9

Even rappers don't have a rhythm like this.

Atrial fibrillation is very important clinically. It can be a sign in a patient who has just had surgery that he or she has had a *pulmonary embolism* or clot in his or her lungs, which unless diagnosed very quickly, can be fatal. If the atrial fibrillation persists it can lead to the patient developing a clot in his left atrium which can travel to the arteries of his brain and cause a stroke.

If you look directly at the heart of a patient with atrial fibrillation you will see at once the atria are contracting like a bag of worms. There are little contractions everywhere. There is no organized contraction. Because of that blood pools in the large left atrium and clots.

The EKG shows irregularly spaced but totally normal QRS complexes and T waves. There aren't any P waves. Sometimes the baseline is totally flat while sometimes it shows tiny irregular waves.

Treatment is two-fold. If the onset of the atrial fibrillation is recent, the patient can be cardioverted electrically. If it has been present for a while, generally more than two days, the patient should first be placed on anticoagulants to prevent clotting and then after a few weeks cardioverted.

If the patient is older he or she can be left on anticoagulants indefinitely. While the atria do contribute a little to the cardiac output, normally about 20%, unless the person is very active, he or she will not notice the dysrhythmia.

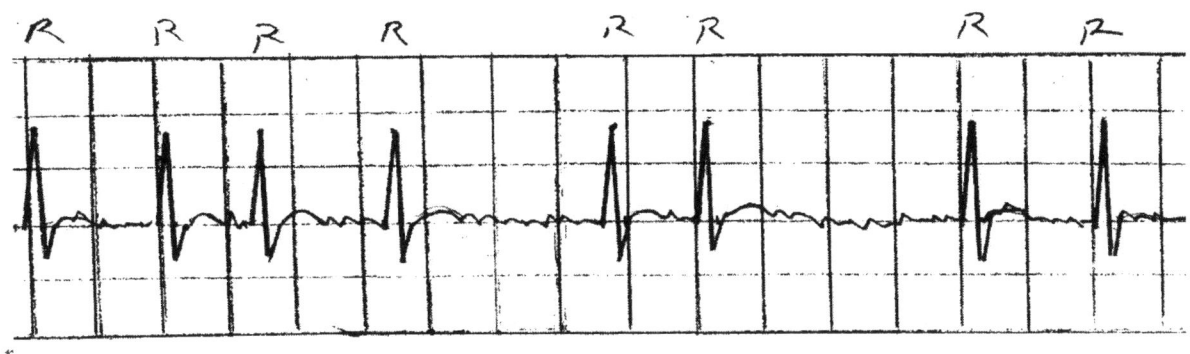

The rhythm is chaotic. There is no pattern at all. But the QRS complexes are totally normal.

The most important thing to remember about atrial fibrillation is its relationship with a pulmonary embolism. You must always check your patient's pulse before you give a treatment of any kind to the patient. If the pulse has always been regular but is now irregularly irregular it is imperative that you let the nurses and doctors know at once. It could very well be a matter of life and death.

Multifocal Atrial Tachycardia (MAT) is characterized by the presence of a chaotic rhythm with at least three different types of P waves, each with its own PR interval. The QRS complexes appear normal. MAT is almost always due to severe lung disease such as chronic obstructive lung disease. However, hypoxemia, theophylline toxicity, and acute coronary artery disease syndromes such as angina can also cause it. It is treated differently from other atrial arrhythmias. It responds best to calcium channel blockers such as Diltiazem or Cardizem as well as to the treatment of the underlying pulmonary condition.

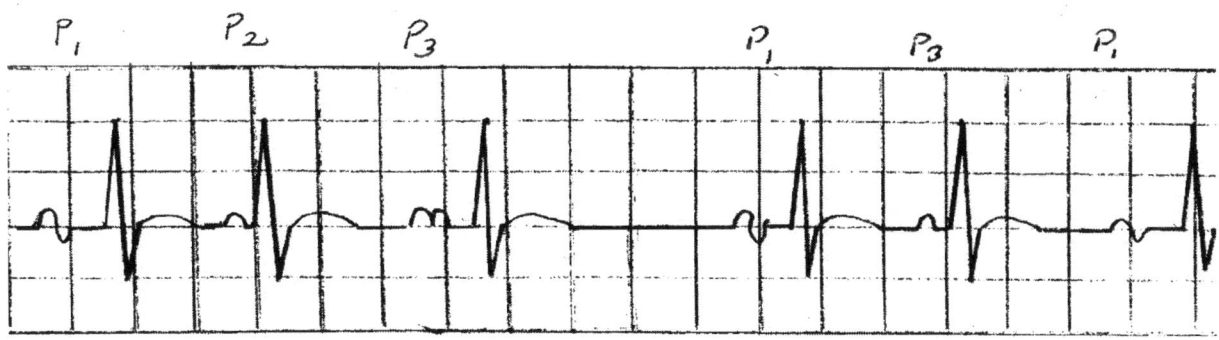

Multifocal Atrial Tachycardia.

The rhythm is irregularly irregular and there are three different types of P waves, each with their own PR interval.

Ventricular *Arrhythmias*

The last set of dysrhythmias is the **ventricular arrhythmias**. There are only three we need to be concerned about. The first is *Premature Ventricular Contractions (PVC)*, the second is *Ventricular Tachycardia (VT)* and the third is *Ventricular Fibrillation (VF)*.

Premature Ventricular Contractions are fairly common and may or may not indicate serious disease. They are caused by an abnormal electrical focus in one of the ventricles. The signal from the focus moves swiftly through the ventricles but can't be transmitted back to the atria because of the one-way channel in the AV node and Bundle of His. Thus the SA node continues to fire regularly. Thusly, after a PVC there is a long "compensatory pause".

The EKG appearance of a PVC is typical. The P wave is absent. The QRS is broad and deformed. If there is only one ectopic focus then all the PVC's appear the same. If there are two ectopic foci, there will be two different types of PVC's on the EKG tracing. The T wave will be inverted and the segment between the end of the S wave and beginning of the T wave will be depressed.

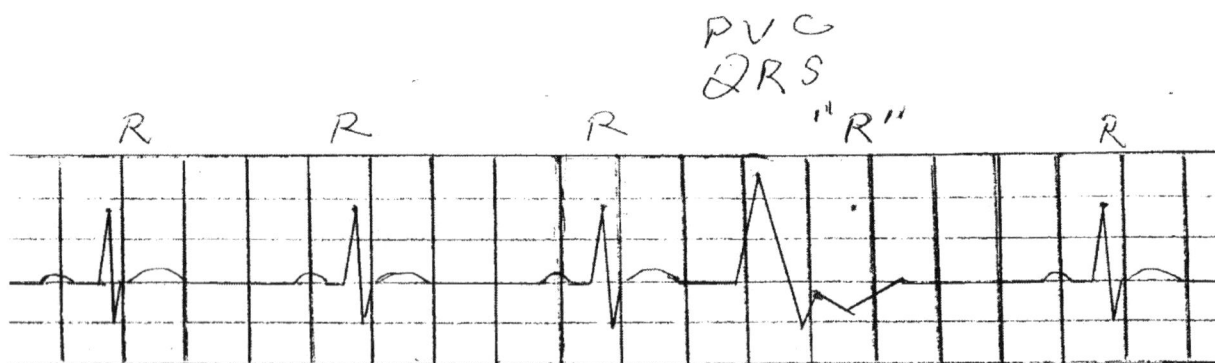

Premature Ventricular Contraction

The fourth beat is a single PVC. The distance from the R preceding the PVC to the R following the PVC is exactly two normal beats. There is a full compensatory pause.

One occasional PVC is of little concern. But three PVC's in a row is a different kind of story altogether. Three or more PVC's in a row is *Ventricular Tachycardia* which is often a fatal arrhythmia.

Ventricular Tachycardia is characterized by serial PVC's. The heart rate is usually between 70 and 100 but may be faster. The patient is usually pulseless but some patients are actually alert, at least for a while. It always indicates serious cardiac disease and must be treated, preferentially with immediate defibrillation.

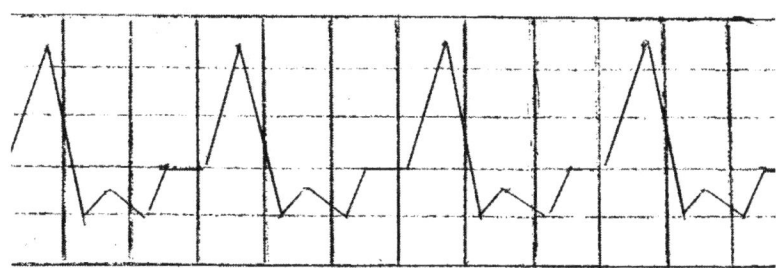

Slow Ventricular Tachycardia with a Heart Rate of 100

Surprisingly this patient may actually be alert.

Ventricular Fibrillation is a fatal arrhythmia. The patient is unresponsive, cyanotic, and usually gasping for air. There is no pulse or blood pressure. If you could see the heart it would look like it is filled with worms crawling about. The EKG shows bizarre giant wave after wave without any semblance of order. The waves are chaotic. Immediate defibrillation must be done or the patient will die.

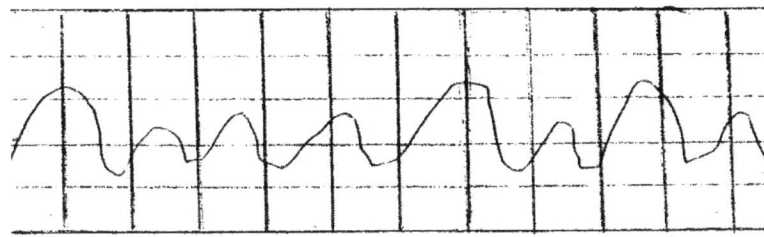

Ventricular Fibrillation

Ventricular Asystole is just that. The patient appears similar to the patient with Ventricular Fibrillation but the EKG shows only a flat line. The heart is dead. Beta adrenergic agents, such as *epinephrine*, are given to try to stimulate the heart to contract but the situation is grim.

One last "arrhythmia" must be mentioned. In this situation there is *electro-mechanical dissociation*. The EKG appears normal or near normal because the electrical pathways are intact but there is no pulse or blood pressure because the heart muscle can't contract. The patient appears, and is for all practical points, dead. Again, Beta adrenergic agents such as epinephrine can be given in an effort to stimulate the heart muscle but they are usually of little avail.

Heart Block

Sometimes communication between the atria and ventricles is impaired. This generally occurs if the signal from the SA node is blocked at the AV node. The P wave and QRS complexes appear normal on the EKG. The blockage at the AV node can be mild. In first degree A-V block, there is a prolonged PR interval between the beginning of the P wave and the beginning of the QRS. Care must be taken before making this diagnosis as the PR interval increases as the heart slows. If the heart rate is 60 a PR interval of .24 seconds is normal while if the heart rate were 80, the same PR interval of .24 would be abnormal.

As the block between the atria and ventricle increases, the relationship between the P waves and QRS complexes deteriorates. There are two types of second degree block. In one type, the P waves appear normal as do the PR intervals, but every few beats there is a P wave without a QRS. This is called Mobitz Type 2. It is as if the conduction is totally blocked every few beats. The other type of second degree heart block is more fascinating. The PR interval gets longer and longer until finally the beat is dropped. This is called the Wenckebach Phenomenon or Mobitz Type 1 Heart Block.

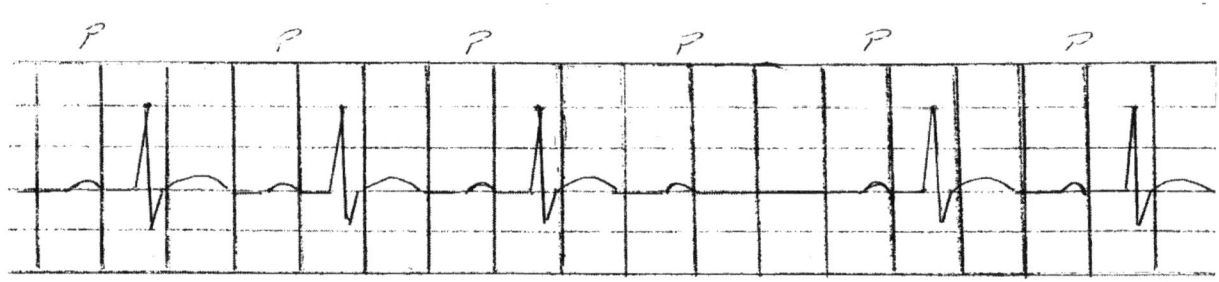

Mobitz Type 2: Each P wave has a QRS and the PR interval is constant until the fourth P wave when the QRS is blocked.

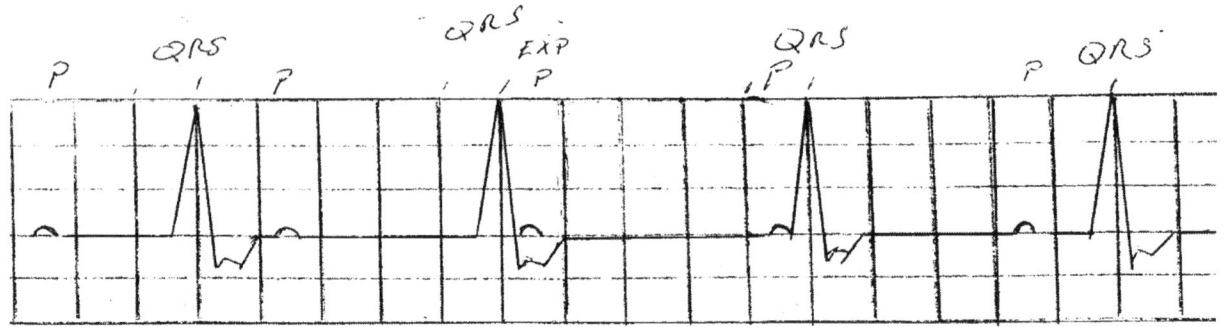

Mobitz Type 1 with progressive prolongation of the PR interval until the QRS complex is lost. The P wave is buried in the QRS.

Complete heart block occurs when the communication between the atria and ventricles is totally disrupted. Surprisingly this can often be difficult to see on an EKG tracing. Basically, the P waves appear normal and have their own rate while the ventricles appear normal and have their own rate. Each is going about his own business, totally ignoring the other.

Lecture Notes: Anatomy and Physiology for the Respiratory Therapist

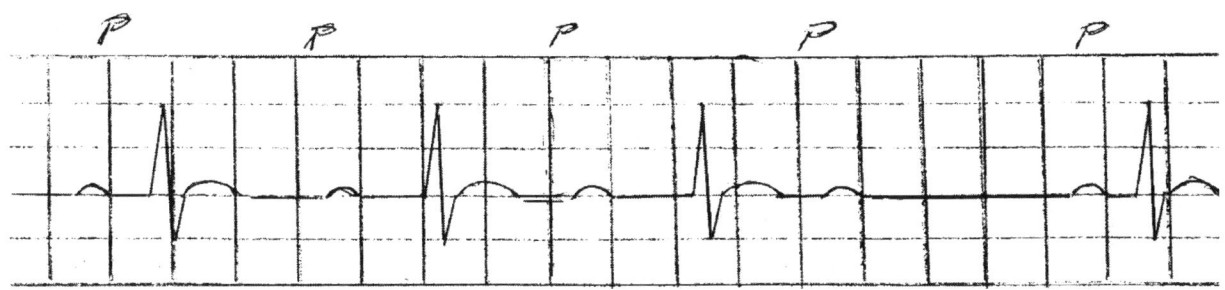

Complete Heart Block.

The atria have their own rate (100) and the ventricles have their own rate (75)

The last "arrhythmia" we need to look at is the "pacemaker artifact". When the pacemaker fires there will be a very thin "spike" on the EKG tracing followed by a bizarre QRS. The rate will be a fixed, usually about 70 to 80 depending on the pacemaker setting. P waves may or may not be present.

IMPORTANT CONCEPTS TO REMEMBER FROM THIS LECTURE

1. Atrial fibrillation is:
   - Characterized by an irregularly irregular rhythm
   - May be the presenting finding of a pulmonary embolism

2. Multifocal Atrial Tachycardia is
   - An irregular rhythm; the EKG shows at least 3 different shaped P waves and PR intervals; it is most commonly associated with severe COPD

3. Third degree heart block is characterized by:
   - No relationship between the atria and ventricles on the EKG. The atria and ventricles each beat at their own rate.

Lecture 5

Putting it All Together

Now that we understand the electrical circuitry and the anatomy of the heart including the heart chambers and heart valves, we can describe the events that occur during a contraction of the heart. The following graft combines the EKG (the bottom of the graft), the pressure changes that occur, first in the atria, then in the ventricles (the top of the graft), and the sounds we hear with our stethoscope as the heart contracts (the middle line). The graph allows us to relate the pressure changes in the heart to the opening and closing of the heart valves.

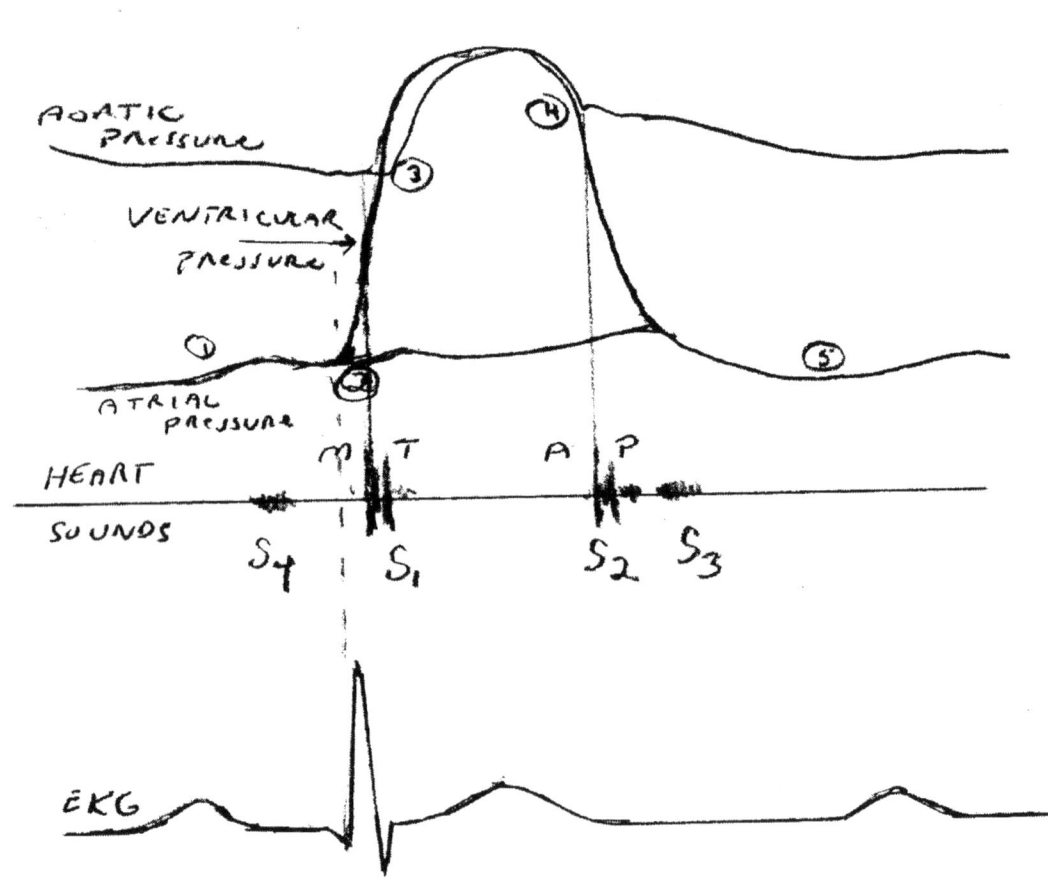

The Relationship between EKG, Heart Sounds, and pressures in the atria and ventricles.

The seemingly complex drawing above gathers everything you know about the heart and puts it in one place. When the P wave or atrial excitation begins the pressure in the atria start to rise (circle 1). At this point, the pressure in the atria becomes higher than the pressure in the ventricles. . Blood rushes into the ventricles from the atria as the atria contract and we sometimes hear a sound, called an S4. In patients with a "stiff" left ventricle due to hypertension, the S4 can be quite loud. It is best heard at the apex of the heart.

When the electrical signal crosses the AV node and the ventricle begins to depolarize as shown by the presence of the QRS complex on the EKG, the pressure in the left ventricle rises abruptly. When the pressure in the ventricles exceeds the pressure in the atria, the mitral and tricuspid valves slam shut (circle 2) and we hear a "lub" sound. This is, of course, S1, or the first heart sound.

The pressure in the ventricles rises abruptly as the heart contracts. When the pressure in the ventricles exceed the pressures in the aorta and pulmonary artery, the aortic and pulmonary valves open (circle 3) and blood flows from both ventricles into both arteries.

As the ventricular contraction peaks and then relaxes, the pressure in the ventricles falls. When the pressure in the ventricles is less than the pressure in the aorta and pulmonary artery, the aortic and pulmonic valves close (circle 4) and we hear the "dub". This is the second heart sound or S2.

The pressure in the ventricles continues to fall and when the ventricular pressure is low enough the mitral and tricuspid valve open. There is an inrushing of blood from the atria into the ventricles and we sometimes hear an S3 or third heart sound. Again, this is best heard at the apex of the heart.

When the heart is at rest, the mitral valve is open. Therefore the pressure in the left atrium and the left ventricle is the same. This pressure is called the *diastolic pressure* and is an important physiologic measurement. The diastolic pressure is a measure of the diastolic volume.

Definitions

There are several terms we need to keep in mind. The first two are systole and diastole. Systole is a term describing ventricular contraction. Diastole is the relaxed heart.

Stroke Volume is the amount of blood in cc's that the heart ejects with each beat. It is usually about 70 cc's. The *cardiac output* is the stroke volume multiplied by the heart rate. If we have a student at rest with a stroke volume of 70 cc's and a heart rate of 72 his cardiac output is about 5,000 cc's.

But the left ventricle does not eject all the blood it contains with every beat. The heart ejects only a fraction of that amount. The volume of blood when the left ventricle is at rest in diastole is about 120 cc. So the *left ventricular ejection fraction (LVEF)* is:

LVEF = amount of blood ejected/diastolic volume

LVEF = 70 cc/120 cc or 58%

The LVEF is one of the most important measurements of cardiac function. We will encounter it again when we discuss congestive heart failure.

How large the ventricles are at the start of their contraction will determine, at least in part, how hard the heart will contract. The heart is like a rubber band. The longer you stretch it, without breaking it of course, the greater it will spring back. The volume of the heart at diastole is called the *left ventricular end diastolic volume (LVEDV)*. This is also referred to as the *preload.* Not surprisingly, the LVEDV is much more easily evaluated by measuring the *left ventricular end diastolic pressure (LVEDP)*. The greater the end diastolic volume or pressure, the more blood the heart will eject because it contracts more forcefully. Like the rubber band, it has been stretched more. We can get an idea of the *preload* by measuring the *end diastolic pressure* which is directly related to the *end diastolic volume*.

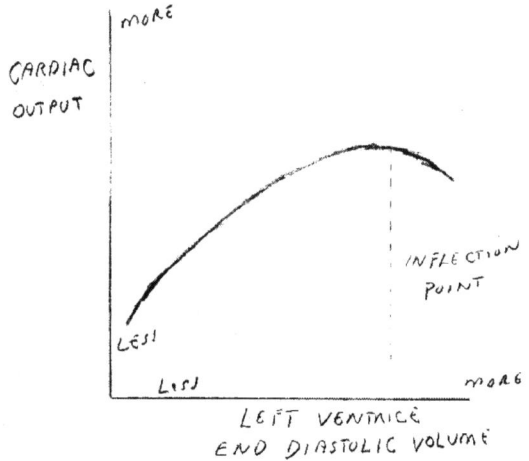

The Relationship between Cardiac Output and the Left Ventricular End Diastolic Volume (LVEDP or LVEDV). The Cardiac Output increases with increasing LVEDV till the inflection point when it suddenly falls off. The heart has been stretched too far!

The left ventricle works directly against the pressure in the aorta. If the pressure in the aorta is high, the left ventricle has to work harder to expel the blood it holds. If the pressure in the aorta is low, the heart doesn't have to work as hard. The force against which the left ventricle, and for that matter the right ventricle, works is called the *Afterload.* The Afterload is directly related to the patient's blood pressure or, in the case of the right ventricle, the pulmonary artery pressure. The higher the blood pressure, the greater the afterload. The greater the *afterload,* the less blood the ventricle will eject.

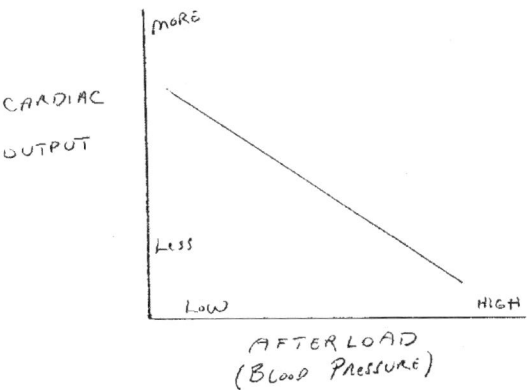

The Relationship between the blood pressure or afterload and the Cardiac Output.

The last concept is that of *contractility.* The heart can contract forcefully or weakly. How much force the heart uses is called its *contractility*.

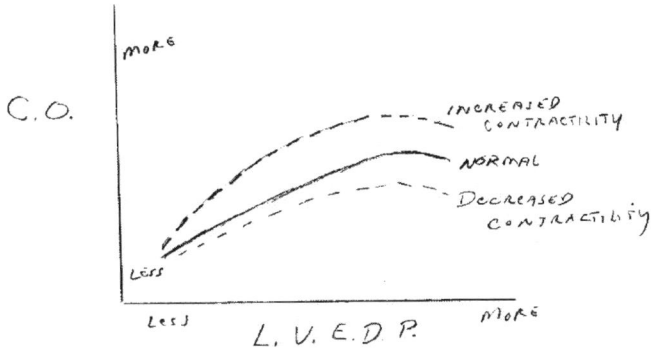

Contractility is the force exerted by the left ventricle during systole.

Some of the medicines we use directly affect the contractility. For example, Beta adrenergic agents, such as epinephrine or albuterol, increase the contractility while Beta Blockers such as Toprol and Propranolol, both common blood pressure medications, reduced the contractility. Digoxin, a heart medicine rarely used nowadays, increases contractility as does the Thyroid hormone.

Common Heart Conditions

The two most common cardiac diseases are **coronary artery disease** and **hypertension**.

Coronary artery disease is due to blockage of the coronary arteries, the arteries which supply oxygen to the heart muscle, and is caused by atherosclerosis or "hardening of the arteries". The blockage is due to the buildup of plaque which is made up of fat, clot, and calcium. Coronary artery disease usually presents as either chest pain or shortness of breath.

The chest pain is due to ischemia of the heart muscle caused by a blockage of a coronary artery. It can take one of two forms. The first type is called *angina*. The patient with angina has chest pain, usually a pressure or squeezing pain in the center of his chest which sometimes runs down his left arm to his elbow. The pain occurs when the patient exerts himself or is under stress. The pain is due to the partial blockage of one of the coronary arteries. At rest, the heart distal to the blockage gets enough oxygen, but with exercise the heart races and as it races, the time for filling of the coronary arteries decreases as diastole decreases and so the muscle fails to get the oxygen it needs and the patient has pain. As soon as the patient stops exercising his heart slows, allowing more time for filling of the coronary arteries, and the pain goes away.

The other type of pain occurs when a plaque in a coronary artery ruptures and fatty substance is released completely blocking the artery. This is called a *myocardial infarction* or a heart attack. The pain is similar to angina but often occurs at rest and does not go away. With every passing minute more and more heart tissue dies from lack of oxygen. Treatment must be started as soon as possible to preserve as much heart muscle as possible. The patient should be given Aspirin immediately. The patient needs to have a heart catherization and have the clot removed and the artery opened up as soon as possible to minimize the damage to the heart.

Coronary artery disease can also present as shortness of breath due to congestive heart failure. In this condition, the heart has suffered many small heart attacks and the heart muscle has become weak. The heart loses its *contractility* or its ability to contract forcefully. When the heart is no longer able to pump enough blood to supply the body's tissues with oxygen and other nutrients the patient has congestive heart failure. This type of congestive heart failure is called *systolic heart failure*.

When the cardiac output falls, the kidneys get less blood. They react by retaining more salt and water. This causes fluid to build up in the great veins. The buildup of fluid increases the *preload* or left ventricular end diastolic volume (usually measured as the left ventricular end diastolic pressure) allowing the left ventricle to fill with more blood and become larger during diastole and thus able to pump a little more blood during systole. But this only helps for a short time. When the *preload* increases to the point where the slope of the contractility exceeds its peak value, like the rubber band stretched too far, the cardiac output falls instead of rising. The left ventricular ejection fraction (LVEF) falls dramatically. The patient's blood pressure falls, the kidneys fail, the patient has even more edema in his or her feet, and the patient becomes anxious, confused, and diaphoretic.

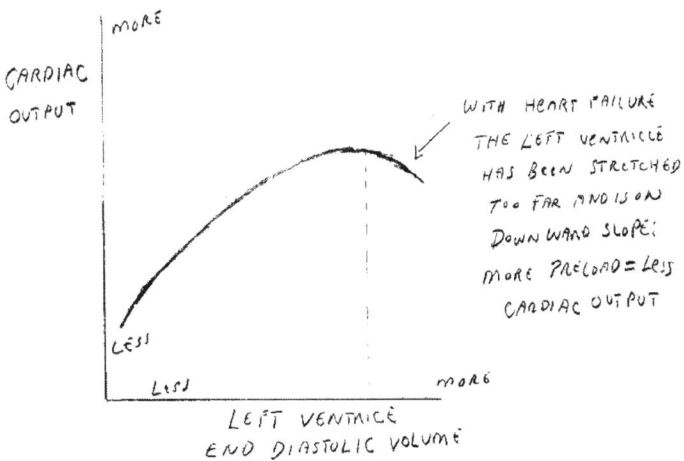

The treatment of congestive heart failure is to decrease the preload by getting rid of the fluid by giving the patient a diuretic such as furosemide as well as to improve contractility with a Beta Adrenergic agent such as Dobutamide or Epinephrine. If the patient's blood pressure is adequate the patient may also be treated with *afterload* reduction by using an *Angiotensin Converting Enzyme Inhibitor* such as Captopril or an *Angiotensin Receptor Blocker* such as Diovan.

Hypertension is "high blood pressure". The normal blood pressure is 120/80 or less. As the pressure increases above 140/90 the heart has to work harder to pump blood. The average or mean blood pressure is the *afterload* against which the heart works.

Like the weight lifter who lifts heavier and heavier weights in order to develop large biceps and triceps, as the heart works harder and harder to overcome the *afterload,* the walls of the left ventricle will become thicker and more muscular. The blood volume in the left ventricle during diastole will become smaller and smaller. The heart will pump less and less blood with each heart beat and the cardiac output will fall. But the Left Ventricular Ejection Fraction is normal. The brain, kidneys, and other tissues of the body will get less and less oxygen and nutrients. This type of heart failure is called *diastolic heart failure.*

The treatment of diastolic heart failure is to lower the *afterload* by reducing the blood pressure.

Heart Murmurs in General

Heart murmurs result from vibrations set up in the blood stream and the surrounding heart and great vessels as a result of turbulent blood flow. The two most common heart murmurs seen in the adult patient are *mitral insufficiency* in which the mitral valve has become leaky and *aortic valve stenosis* in which the aortic valve has become stiff and its opening narrowed.

How can you diagnose a heart murmur?

The first step in evaluating a heart murmur is to determine if the murmur occurs in systole or diastole. Mitral insufficiency and aortic stenosis both occur during systole. Next, determine where the murmur is best heard. The aortic murmurs are heard best in the second intercostal space to the right of the sternum. Mitral murmurs are heard at the apex of the heart. The third step is to listen carefully and determine the characteristics of the murmur. Does the murmur wax and wane? This is called a *Crescendo-Decrescendo* murmur and is characteristic of aortic stenosis. Or is the murmur constant? This is called a *plateau* murmur or if it occurs in systole a *holosystolic murmur* and is characteristic of mitral insufficiency. Lastly, how loud is the murmur? Do you have to strain to hear the murmur? This is a grade 1 murmur. Or can you feel the murmur with your hand gently placed over the heart. This is called a *thrill* or palpable murmur and makes the murmur a grade 4 murmur.

Systolic Murmurs

There are four common systolic murmurs. The most common is the murmur of Mitral Insufficiency or Mitral Regurgitation. The function of the mitral valve is to prevent blood from leaking back into the left atrium when the left ventricle contracts. If the valve is leaky, as the left ventricle contracts blood will squirt back into the left atrium. Since the pressure in the left ventricle is higher than the left atrium throughout systole, the murmur will begin with the first heart sound, which will be soft, and engulf the second heart sound. The murmur sounds like a "swoosh" and is constant in pitch and intensity. It is thus "holosystolic". It is heard best at the apex of the heart.

The most common cause of mitral regurgitation is an extremely dilated left ventricle. The valve just can't close the valvular opening completely. Another common cause is when one of the supporting struts of the valve has been damaged by a heart attack. The remaining struts can't close the valve completely. The murmur can also be due to endocarditis or infection of the endocardium lining the valve. The treatment is surgical. The valve must be replaced.

A variant of mitral regurgitation is the *"click-murmur"* syndrome also known as *mitral valve prolapse*. This is a fairly common disorder of young women who are thin with very straight backs. In fact for some time, it was called the *straight back syndrome*. The auscultatory findings are classic. There is a loud, mid-systolic, metallic sounding, "click", followed by a short high pitched murmur which waxes and wanes. I like to imagine the chordae tendoneae "suddenly stretched tightly" causing the click, followed by a little leak which causes the murmur.

Mitral Valve Prolapse is generally a "non-problem". Most people outgrow the murmur. Sometimes, however, it is associated with asthma and chest pain caused by inflammation of the costochondral cartilages called "costochondritis". Rarely, the syndrome is associated with premature ventricular contractions and even more rarely with an infection in the mitral valve called *endocarditis*.

Aortic Stenosis commonly occurs as patients grow older. The aortic valve becomes calcified and stiffens. It becomes harder and harder for blood to squeeze through the narrowed valve from the left ventricle to the aorta. It can also occur if the patient was born with a bicuspid valve instead of the normal tricuspid valve. In other words, there are two cusps instead of the normal three. The murmur is classic. It is best heard in the second interspace to the right of the sternum. It begins when the aortic valve opens, after the first heart sound, and increases in intensity as the left ventricle contracts and then as the left ventricle relaxes it wanes in intensity. It is thus a *"crescendo-decrescendo" murmur*.

The patient usually presents with chest pain because the left ventricular wall becomes thickened and requires more oxygen. The treatment is always a valve replacement but now the new valve can be replaced through a transcatheter approach (TAVR or transcatheter aortic valve replacement) done via heart catheterization rather than with open heart surgery.

About 30% of older adults will have a normal aortic valve even though they have a murmur of aortic stenosis.

Lastly, in newborns and infants, the pulmonary artery may be congenitally narrowed or the pulmonary valve may have two leaflets which are partially fused instead of the normal freely moving three leaflets. In either case the infant is short of breath with signs of right heart failure including edema of the feet. The auscultatory findings are classic. Like aortic stenosis, there is a crescendo-decrescendo murmur which is best heard at the second interspace to the left of the sternum.

Pulmonary artery stenosis is found with other congenital defects such as the *Tetralogy of Fallot*. The treatment is surgical.

Diastolic Murmurs

Diastolic murmurs are very uncommon. The most frequent diastolic murmurs are aortic regurgitation due to a leaky aortic valve, and mitral stenosis due to a narrowed mitral valve.

Aortic regurgitation is due to a leaky valve allowing blood to flow backwards from the aorta into the left ventricle as the heart muscle relaxes. The most common cause is *Marfan's Syndrome*, which is a genetic disorder that affects the connective tissue. The patient is tall, lean, long-armed and legged, double-jointed, and often has visual problems. Some doctors think that Abe Lincoln had Marfan's Syndrome, but of course, we will never know for sure. Aortic regurgitation can also be seen in a patient with syphilis.

The murmur begins after the second heart sound and is decrescendo, like a "wisp". Unlike aortic stenosis which is best heard in the 2nd right intercostal space, the murmur of aortic regurgitation is heard best in the third left intercostal space, which is also known as Erb's point. This probably occurs because the direction of the blood flow is from the aorta towards the apex of the left ventricle. Having the patient sit up and lean forward is helpful. Because of the leak, the left ventricle enlarges and the patient develops congestive heart failure. He becomes short of breath. The treatment is surgical. The surgery needs to be done within a year after the onset of symptoms.

Mitral stenosis is now quite rare. It is unlikely you will ever see a patient with the disorder. It was quite common a hundred years ago when Rheumatic Fever was a common disease. The development of Penicillin probably ended the epidemic. The murmur is best described as a low-pitched "rumble" which occurs just before the first heart sound.

In the past, when rheumatic fever was common, heart disease due to mitral stenosis was frequently seen. The patients presented with shortness of breath and a very large heart, and because blood backed up into the lungs, they often had hemoptysis and even pulmonary fibrosis. The treatment was to dilate the valve using a catheter or to replace the valve.

Congenital Heart Disease

Heart defects in fetuses are quite common. Between 10 and 20% of fetuses have heart defects but most of the fetuses with heart defects are still borne or miscarried.

The two most common heart defects in children are a ventricular septal defect (VSD) and a bicuspid aortic valve, both of which occur in about 3% of newborns. Most of the VSD's close within a year of life. Bicuspid aortic valvular disease often presents in the 60's and 70's because of the development of aortic stenosis.

Besides these two disorders, about 1% of newborns will have a serious heart defect including left to right shunts, right to left shunts, or an obstructive lesion such as pulmonary artery stenosis.

There are three types of left to right shunts. They are named based on the location of the shunt. The shunt can be due to a hole in the atria called an *atrial septal defect (ASD)*, a hole in the ventricle called a *ventricular septal defect (VSD)*, or a connection between the aorta and the pulmonary artery called a *Patent Ductus Arteriosus (PDA)*. In all of these defects the baby may be asymptomatic at birth because blood flows normally from the right side of the heart into the lungs, where it is oxygenated, and then to the left side of the heart. Most of the blood on the left side of the heart leaves the heart normally but some of the blood escapes back through the defect in the heart back to the right side of the heart. Over time the right side of the heart hypertrophies because of the extra blood it receives due to the shunting and the shunt becomes a right to left shunt. The child will then become cyanotic, first with exercise and then even at rest. This is called the *Eisenmenger's Syndrome*. The treatment is surgical.

The type of murmur heard depends upon the type of defect. With an ASD, the murmur is typically like that of pulmonary artery stenosis. With a VSD the murmur is systolic in timing, loud, harsh, and to the left of the sternum at about the 4th or 5th interspace. With a PDA, the murmur is best described as "machinery-like" and is best heard over the upper back of the infant.

Of special importance, an ASD may first present in an adult. I have seen a patient with ASD present in her sixties!

There are two major causes of right to left shunts. The first is the *Transposition of the Great Vessels* in which the aorta arises from the right ventricle and the pulmonary artery arises from the left ventricle. This condition is always associated with an ASD or VSD. The second condition is *The Tetralogy of Fallot* which is characterized by a large VSD, Pulmonary Artery Stenosis, Right Ventricular Hypertrophy, and an "overriding" aorta (the aorta arises from both the right and left ventricle). These patients are cyanotic from birth and the treatment is always surgical. They are cyanotic because the blood goes from the right side of the heart to the left side of the heart bypassing the lungs. In the case of the transposition of the great vessels, blood travels from the vena cava to the right atrium to the right ventricle and thence to the aorta. It is only because of the ASD or VSD that any blood gets oxygenated at all. In the case of the Tetralogy blood flows from the vena cava to the right atrium and thence the right ventricle and then some of the blood goes to the lungs and some of the blood goes to the aorta. Again, only the VSD allows the blood to get any oxygen.

Coarctation of the Aorta is a narrowing or constriction of a portion of the thoracic aorta. It is much more common in men than in women. Symptoms include headaches, nosebleeds, cold extremities, and intermittent claudication (pain in a muscle with exercise). The hallmark finding is that the blood pressure is higher in the arms than in the legs, the exact opposite of what you would normally expect. The pulses in the feet are barely palpable. There is also a mid-systolic murmur heard over the back. Notching of the ribs is often seen on the chest x-ray. The treatment is surgical.

IMPORTANT CONCEPTS TO REMEMBER FROM THIS LECTURE

1. What is Afterload?

   – The force against which the heart must contract. Essentially, it is the mean arterial blood pressure.

2. What is Preload?

   – The size of the left ventricle during diastole, when the heart is relaxed, or the left ventricular end diastolic volume.

3. What percentage of fetuses have heart defects?

   – 10-20% of fetuses.

4. What percentage of adults over 65 will have a murmur of aortic stenosis with a normal aortic valve?

   – About 30%.

Lecture Six

The Circulation

How many ventricles do we really need?

Do all creatures have two atria and two ventricles? Why use nearly twice as much nutrients, such as oxygen, to support two ventricles? Why not just have one ventricle? Fish have only one atrium and one ventricle. Blood enters the heart through the atrium and is passed to the ventricle. When the ventricle contracts blood is forced out through the capillaries of the gills and then collected and distributed to the rest of the fish's body. This sounds more efficient to me!

Amphibians and reptiles go one step beyond the fish. Frogs have two atria but only one ventricle. One atrium receives oxygenated blood from the lungs while the other receives deoxygenated blood from the organs. The atria then send their blood to the ventricle. However, the ventricle has a membrane that divides it effectively in half so that when it contracts oxygenated blood goes to the organs of the body and deoxygenated blood goes to the lungs.

Crocodiles are the exception. They have four chambers just like birds and mammals. What is the advantage of four chambers?

The four-chambered system allows for two types of circulation. One circulation uses large-bore, thick-walled, high-pressure blood vessels to transport blood from one of the ventricles of the heart to the organs of the body. Imagine the force needed to transport blood from the heart of a giraffe up to its brain. That's a distance of seven or eight feet and sometimes even more.

On the other hand, the circulation going to the lungs is able to use thin-walled, stretchable tubing since the heart has to pump the blood to a height of no more than a few inches. Just look at your chest wall. The heart sits directly behind the sternum. The pulmonary artery is behind the Angle of Louis, the little ridge of the sternum you feel as you run your hand up the bone. The apex of the lung is just behind your clavicle. The distance between the origin of the pulmonary artery and the top of your lungs is no more than a few inches.

When the right ventricle contracts it fills and distends the very flexible pulmonary arteries so that when the pulmonary valve closes as the heart enters diastole, these stretched arteries continue to squeeze blood through the capillaries of the lung as they relax due to elastic recoil. Thus, instead of the lung's capillaries getting blood just during systole when the heart contracts, a mere $1/3^{rd}$ of the time, the capillaries get blood all the time, allowing for more efficient transport of oxygen from the alveoli to the blood.

That's why we are better off than frogs.

The Circulation in General

The aorta arises directly from the left ventricle. As it arches across the top of the heart from the right side of the mediastinum to the left before taking a descending course, the aorta sends three branches supplying the head and neck and arms. The first is the *brachiocephalic artery* which branches into the *right subclavian artery* and the *right common carotid artery*. The second is the *left common carotid artery*, and finally the third branch is the *left subclavian artery*. The common carotid arteries divide into an *external carotid artery* which supplies the tissues of the head and neck and the *internal carotid arteries* which supply the brain. The internal carotid arteries actually pass through the little groove located between the pillars guarding the tonsillar tissue at the sides of your throat. Like your mother said, "Don't run around with a pencil in your mouth! If you fall you'll have a stroke" Mothers are always right!

The aorta then passes downward through the chest giving off branches to the trachea and major airways of the lungs, called the *bronchial arteries*. We sometimes believe that the lungs get their nutrients from the pulmonary arteries but that is just not the case. Most of the bronchi, large and small, get their oxygen and other nutrients from the bronchial arteries.

After the aorta passes through the diaphragm it sends branches to the kidneys, the *Renal Arteries*, and then branches to the gut, the *Superior and Inferior Mesenteric Arteries*. As the aorta enters the pelvis it divides into the *Iliac Arteries*, which then continue into the thighs as the *Femoral Arteries* and the calves as the *Popliteal Arteries* finally ending in the feet dividing into the *Dorsalis Pedis Arteries* and the *Posterior Tibial Arteries*.

Each arm is supplied by a *Subclavian Artery* which becomes the *Brachial Artery* after giving off several branches to the chest wall. The brachial artery divides into the *Radial Artery* on the thumb side of your hand and the *Ulnar Artery* on the little finger side of your hand. The two arteries form a plexus of small arteries in the hand so that if either the Radial Artery or Ulnar Artery is blocked the hand will still get oxygenated blood.

The arteries branch into smaller and smaller arterioles and finally into tiny capillaries which are no more than a handful of micrometers in diameter. It is in the capillaries where the blood does its work, supplying tissues with oxygen and nutrients and removing carbon dioxide and waste products. The capillaries draining the tissue reform into larger and larger vessels finally become venules and then ever larger veins till they form the Superior Vena Cava and the Inferior Vena Cava which, together, drain into the right atrium. The systemic circuit is finally complete.

The Pulmonary Circulation begins as the Main Pulmonary Artery exits the right ventricle. It divides almost at once into a left and right main branch. These large branches form part of the hila of the lungs. The branches continue to divide till they form capillaries which surround the alveoli. After passing the alveoli, the capillaries reunite to form larger and larger blood vessels and ultimately the Pulmonary Veins which then enters the left atrium.

The pressures on the right side of the heart are one tenth the pressures on the left side of the heart. If the normal arterial blood pressure is 120/80, the normal peak pressure in the right ventricle is about 12 mm Hg.

The arterial blood pressure depends upon the stroke volume of the left heart as well as the stiffness of the tubing. As with the pulmonary artery, the blood vessels in the arterial circulation are somewhat distensible. The blood pressure is regulated by the *autonomic nervous system* which includes the *sympathetic nervous system* and the *parasympathetic nervous system*.

The sympathetic nervous system is the "fight or flight" nervous system. It is the system which allows us to deal with an acutely stressful situation. Our pupils dilate, our hair stands on end, our heart palpitates, our blood pressure rises, and our bronchi dilate. The blood flow to our brain and muscles increase. However, the blood flow to our gut and kidneys decreases. Who could eat a pizza when they are getting ready for a final exam in physics or when they are being chased by a lion? The primary neurotransmitter for the sympathetic nervous system is epinephrine.

The parasympathetic nervous system, on the other hand, is for a more relaxed time. It helps maintain our normal bowel function. It slows the heart rate. It constricts bronchial smooth muscle. The neurotransmitter is acetylcholine. It is the nervous system for enjoying our pizza.

The autonomic system has several components. The vasomotor center is found in the medulla, the lowest and most primitive part of our brainstem. The output from the vasomotor center is the sympathetic nervous system. The input is supplied by the baroreceptors or pressure receptors found in the Carotid Body and the Aortic Body.

Palpable Pulses

There are several places where the arteries are superficial enough to allow us to be able to feel a pulse. These include the Carotid Arteries in the neck located just inside the large sternocleidomastoid muscles, the Radial Arteries in the wrist located directly above the middle of the index finger, the Ulnar Arteries in the wrist directly above the middle of the ring finger, the Femoral Arteries in the groins, the Dorsalis Pedis Arteries on the top of the foot, and lastly, the Posterior Tibial Arteries on the medial surface of the foot halfway between the Achilles tendon and the large bone called the Medial Malleolus.

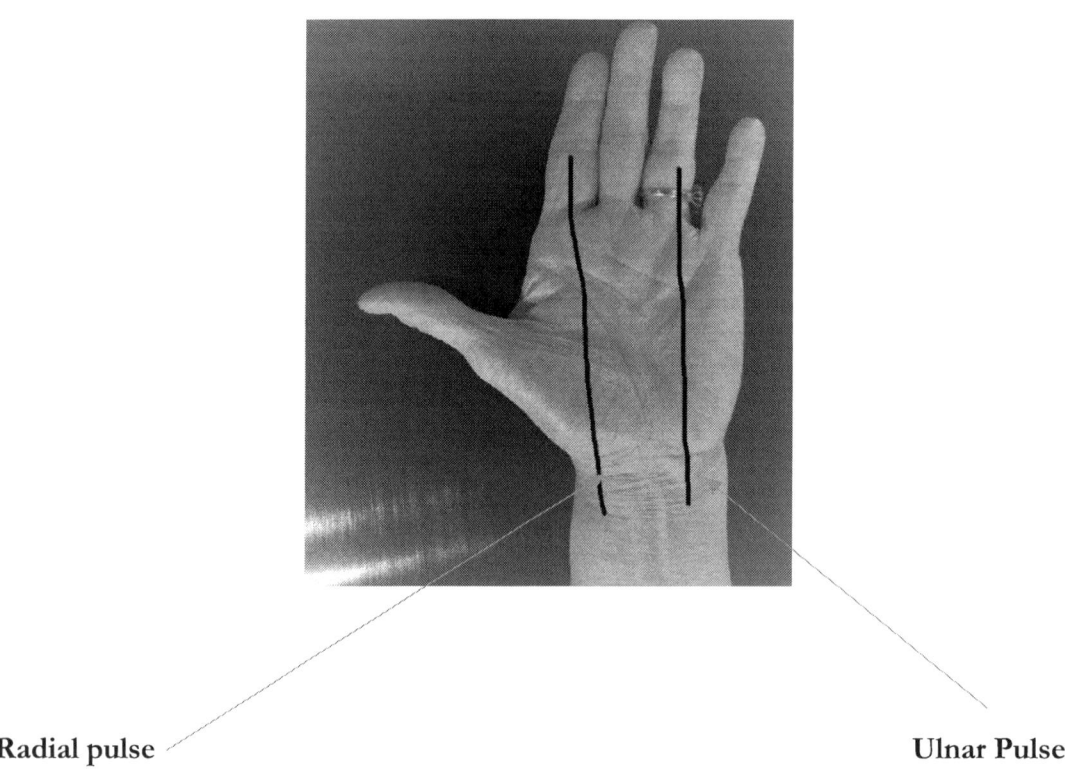

Radial pulse   Ulnar Pulse

Lecture Notes: Anatomy and Physiology for the Respiratory Therapist

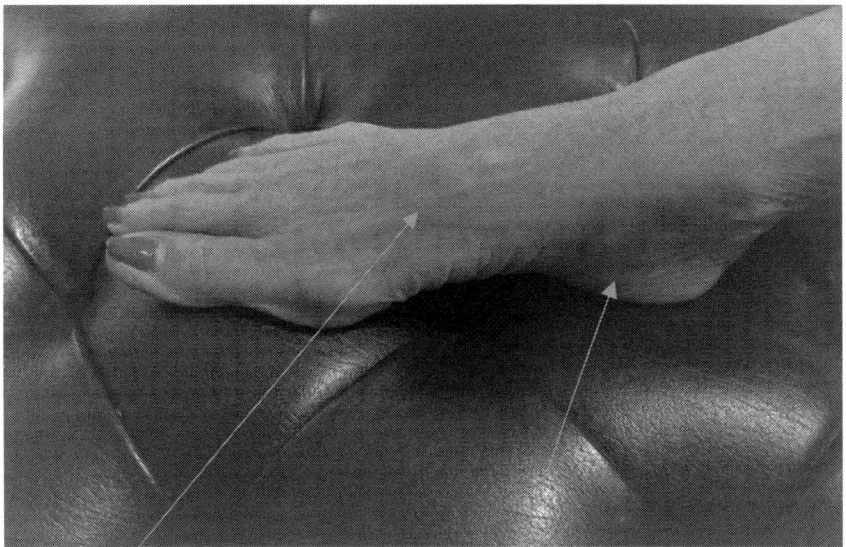

Dorsal Pedis Pulse   **Posterior Tibial Pulse**

It is important to make sure that the ulnar artery is patent before drawing a blood gas from the radial artery. The modified Allen test is performed as followed. The hand is elevated. The patient is asked to clench his or her fist for about 30 seconds. Pressure is applied over the ulnar and the radial arteries occluding both of them. While still elevated, the hand is opened and the pressure over the ulnar artery is released. If the Ulnar Artery is patent, the hand should fill with blood and become pink.

Ohm's Law and Poiseuille's Law

We should all recall from high school Ohm's law. I remember it easiest because the equation V = IR is the Latin for "man". Ohm's Law describes mathematically the relationship between the flow of electron or current in a wire (I), the force which makes the electron or current move (V), and the resistance of the wiring through which the current moves (R):

$$V = I \times R$$

Where V is the voltage of a battery, I is the current or flow of electrons and R is the resistance.

From Ohm's Law we derive Poiseuille's (*pronounced PWAAZ EE*) Law which describes mathematically the relationship between the flow of a liquid or gas in a tube, the force which makes the liquid or gas move, and the resistance of the tubing. It applies not only to the aorta, but also to the trachea and major airways, as well as the tubes we use to intubate the patient.

$$P = F \times R$$

Where P is the pressure gradient, F is the flow of blood or gas, and R is the resistance of the tubing.

The Pressure in Poiseuille's law is the pressure difference between two points, for example, the pressure difference between the Aorta as it leaves the left ventricle and the pressure in the Radial

Artery in your hand.   P is always a pressure gradient. The equation for the resistance is more complex.

$$R = K \times 8 \times \text{Length} / \pi \times radius^4$$

Where R is the resistance and K is a constant

Thus resistance increases if the tubing is longer or if the radius decreases (the radius is in the denominator). The longer the tube the greater the resistance. The narrower the tube the greater the resistance. In fact, cursory inspection of the equation shows that the radius is the most important factor in determining the resistance of a tube. If we transfer our equation for R into the equation for Poiseuille's law and solve for the flow rate (F) we get:

$$F = P \times \pi \times radius^4 / K \times 8 \times \text{Length}$$

Thus the flow rate, how fast the blood flows in the aorta or how fast air flows in the trachea, is largely dependent on the radius. If the radius of the tube doubles the flow will increase $2 \times 2 \times 2 \times 2$ or 2^4 or 16 fold.

Applying Poiseuille's law to our study of the circulation we get:

Cardiac Output = mean arterial pressure/resistance

The cardiac output is already familiar to us as is the concept of resistance. The mean arterial pressure is derived from the following formula:

$$\text{MAP} = (\text{SBP} + (2 \times \text{DPB}))/ 3$$

Where MAP = Mean Arterial Blood Pressure, SBP is the systolic blood pressure and DPB is the diastolic blood pressure.

The MAP is already well known to us. It is the afterload against which the left ventricle must work.

Starling's Law

The circulation in the capillaries is governed by Starling's Law which relates the movement of water into and out of a capillary to the physical and osmotic pressures inside and outside of capillaries.

Capillaries, wherever they are found, are tiny tubes measuring no more than six micrometers in diameter, bounded by a single layer of cells called the endothelium. The capillaries are so small the Red Blood Cells, which measure 7 micra in diameter, must squeeze through them. They are surrounded by interstitial tissue which contains fibrous strands of protein as well as cells of various types.

The blood inside the capillaries exerts a pressure or force against the wall of the capillaries similar to the force water exerts against the side of a pipe through which it is running. On the other hand the interstitial tissue around the capillaries is pushing back against the capillary trying to keep the fluid inside the tiny tube. The second major force is the osmotic force. As you recall, proteins are made up of amino acids which are quite highly charged. The charged amino acids attract water molecules and bind them (an example of Van der Waal's bonding). The tendency of the proteins to attract the water molecules is called the *osmotic pressure*. There are proteins in the blood as well as even more in the interstitial tissues surrounding the capillaries.

Thus we have Starling's Law:

$$J = K(P_C - P_i) + \delta(OP_i - OP_C)$$

Where J is the flux or the transfer of fluid into or out of the capillary, K is the permeability constant, P_C is the capillary pressure pushing fluid out of the capillary, P_i is the interstitial pressure pushing fluid back into the capillary, δ is the osmotic coefficient, usually one, OP_i is the tissue osmotic pressure pulling fluid into the tissue, and OP_C is the capillary osmotic pressure dragging fluid back into the capillaries.

The problem most students have is that they see this equation as static, but it is very dynamic. P_C is much greater on the arterial side of the capillary than on the venous side of the capillary so that there is a tendency on the arterial side for fluid to flood out of the capillaries and into the interstitial tissue. On the venous side P_C is much smaller and capillary osmotic pressure greater because the fluid has become more concentrated as fluid leaves on the arterial side. Both of these changes drag fluid back into the capillary.

For example:

	Arterial Side	Venous side
Pc	30	16
Pi	3	3
OPc	28	28
OPi	8	8
Net outward force	7	-7

Thus, on the arterial side fluid is rushing from the capillary to the interstitium because of the "positive net outward force", while on the venous side fluid is rushing from the interstitial tissue back into the capillary because of the "negative net outward force". This fluid flux probably enhances the transfer of oxygen and nutrients into the tissues and carbon dioxide and waste products out of the system.

At times, the amount of fluid entering the interstitial tissues on the arterial side can exceed what can reenter the capillaries on the venous side. This tends to occur when the pressure on the venous side is high. The excess fluid is then carried off by the lymphatic tissue which drains into the lymph channels and ultimately into the *Thoracic Duct* which finally returns the fluid back into the circulation.

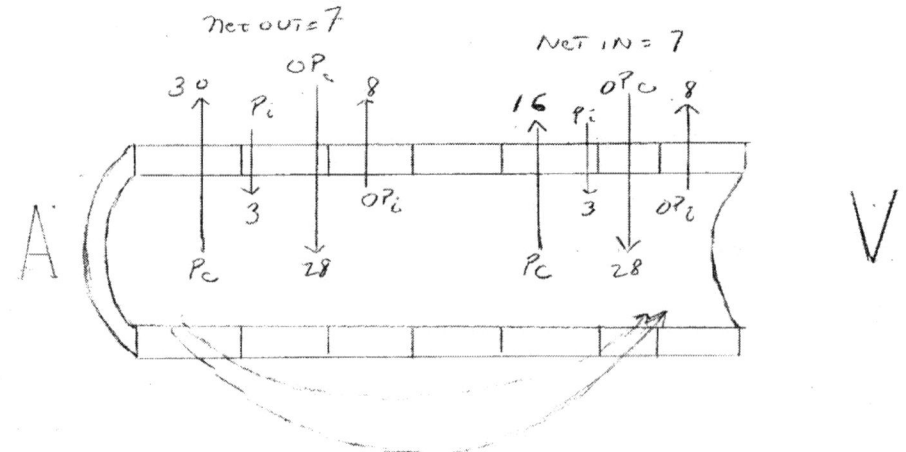

A is the arterial side; V is the venous side

Disorders of the Pulmonary Circulation

The pulmonary circulation is affected by several physiologic factors as well as certain chemicals and medicines. The most important factor is oxygen. If there is a decrease in the alveolar oxygen, an increase in the blood hydrogen ion, or an increase in the alveolar carbon dioxide level, the pulmonary arteries will constrict. The Pulmonary Arterial Resistance will increase placing a strain on the right side of the heart. In addition, epinephrine and other Beta Adrenergic agents will also constrict the pulmonary arteries, unlike the Theophyllines, which dilate them.

Surprisingly, when the right heart stroke volume increases, the pulmonary artery resistance decreases. Likely this is due to the distensibility of the pulmonary artery. The increased fluid volume pushed out by the right ventricle distends the pulmonary artery and because the artery now has a larger radius, the resistance falls. Remember the resistance is inversely related to the fourth power of the radius of the tubing. This factor will result in a better matching of ventilation and perfusion in the alveoli and is likely important in our response to stress and aerobic exercise.

Pathology

The most common acute pathological condition affecting the pulmonary arteries is the *Pulmonary Embolism*. A pulmonary embolism is a blood clot in the lung which has moved or *embolized* from another source, usually a deep vein in the thigh or pelvis. It is especially common in the hospital setting and affects more than a half million Americans every year. 60,000 Americans will die from a pulmonary embolism this year. Yet, if it is diagnosed promptly, the survival rate is 98%.

A thrombus is a clot, composed of a mass of platelets, inflammatory cells, and very a large protein called fibrin, that forms in response to an injury or genetic disorder. The risk of an occurrence of a thrombus is related to Virchow's Triad which is: 1. Hypercoagulability; 2. Injury to the endothelial lining of the blood vessel; and 3. Stasis. Most often, a clot occurs in the large veins of thigh or hip (the femoral vein or iliac vein) in a patient who is hospitalized and at bed rest for a surgery such as a hip replacement or for a medical reason such as congestive heart failure or an exacerbation of chronic lung disease (stasis).

The patient may be hypercoagulable because he has had surgery or trauma. When any blood vessel in the body is injured, the clotting mechanism is activated throughout the entire circulatory system. Thus removing a gallbladder activates the clotting system not only in the abdomen but even in the leg and can cause a clot to form in the thigh. In addition, patients with certain types of cancers including cancers of the prostate, breast, or pancreas are often hypercoagulable. Lastly, certain genetic conditions including deficiencies of certain clotting factors such as Protein C and Protein S, or the presence of Leyden's Factor 5 make the patient more prone to form a clot.

Finally, direct injury to a blood vessel, even something as trivial as being struck by a baseball in the calf, can precipitate a clot.

Most clots simply stay put in the vein and the condition is known as *deep vein thrombosis* but some break apart and chunks of the clot migrate to the lung where they become pulmonary emboli. Some pulmonary emboli are tiny but some can be so large they block both the left and right main pulmonary arteries. This is called a "Saddle Embolus".

There is only one symptom of a pulmonary embolism on which we can hang our hat. 97% of patients with a pulmonary embolism will be short of breath. They may also have chest pain; they may also cough up blood; they may also develop atrial fibrillation and have an irregular pulse. But these other findings occur less than 30% of the time. Because of that, it is imperative that every Respiratory Therapy Practitioner as well as every nurse and doctor be aware that a hospitalized patient who develops the sudden onset of shortness of breath may have a pulmonary embolism. The diagnosis can usually be made with a Helical CAT Scan of the chest. But the diagnosis CAN'T be made unless there is clinical suspicion. Clinical suspicion must come first.

The treatment for a pulmonary embolism depends upon its severity. If the patient is near death, then surgery to remove the clot is the best approach. If the patient is stable, then agents to break up the clot called *fibrinolytics* such as Tissue Plasminogen Activator or Streptokinase should be given along with more traditional blood thinners such as Heparin and Coumadin.

The pulmonary arteries can also be affected chronically in a condition called *chronic pulmonary hypertension*. This is a large group of diseases, some of which are very common, some of which are very rare, but all of which are almost always fatal. In chronic pulmonary hypertension the pressure in the pulmonary arteries rises significantly to well above normal. The normal mean pulmonary artery pressure is less than 20 mm Hg; these patients have a mean pulmonary artery pressure of more than 25 mm Hg at rest and 30 mm Hg with exercise. The rise in the pulmonary artery pressure puts a strain on the right ventricle which ultimately fails and the patient goes into right-sided congestive heart failure.

Chronic Pulmonary Hypertension (PH) is divided into five large groups based on their pathology.

Group 1 is Pulmonary Artery Hypertension (PAH). The idiopathic type of PAH affects mainly young women in the early thirties and is characterized by thickening of the pulmonary artery and its branches. The artery is no longer distensible. The most common symptom is shortness of breath. As the disease progresses the right ventricle hypertrophies and begins to fail, symptoms of congestive heart failure develop. Also included in this group are the collagen vascular disease such as Systemic Lupus Erythematosus and Rheumatoid Arthritis as well as AIDS or the Acquired Immunodeficiency Syndrome due to the HIV (Human Immuno-Virus) and even Schistosomiasis, a disease of the tropics in which the patient is infected by a type of worm. Treatment for this group involves the use of pulmonary arterial dilators such as Sildenafil or Viagra. The gold standard test for making the diagnosis is the right heart catheterization.

Group 2 are those patients who have pulmonary artery hypertension due to left sided heart failure or Congestive Heart Failure. This group accounts for more than 80% of all patients with pulmonary hypertension. The treatment is directed at treating the underlying heart condition.

Group 3 are the patients who have lung disease such as Chronic Obstructive Pulmonary Disease or Obstructive Sleep Apnea. This is the second largest group, accounting for about 10% of patients with pulmonary hypertension. The primary problem in this group is hypoxia. Hypoxia causes Pulmonary Artery constriction and, ultimately, right heart failure. The treatment is directed at both the hypoxia and the lung disease.

Group 4 are patients with *Chronic Thrombo-Embolic Pulmonary Hypertensive Disease (CTEPH)*. These patients have had multiple pulmonary emboli over the years, although even one acute pulmonary embolism that fails to resolve can result in the disorder. The blockage or blockages cause the pressure in the pulmonary artery to rise and the patient to develop right heart failure. The ventilation-perfusion lung scan is more helpful in making this diagnosis than is the helical CAT scan but only if the lung scan is high probability. The treatment is the surgical removal of the clots. The surgery involves bypassing the heart and should be done in a center that specializes in that kind of surgery.

Group 5 are those patients that don't fit into any of the above groups. Some of the patients have Sarcoidosis, some have blood diseases, and some have cancer.

COR PULMONALE

Cor Pulmonale is defined as the abnormal enlargement of the right side of the heart due to lung disease. Most often, it is caused by high pressure in the pulmonary arteries which strain the right ventricle and ultimately cause it to fail. Because of the high prevalence of COPD or chronic obstructive lung disease, cor pulmonale has become much more common. In fact, COPD accounts for 80% of the cases of cor pulmonale in the United Kingdom and more than 50% in the USA. However, any obstructive disease, restrictive disease, or pulmonary vascular disease such as PAH can cause the disorder. A partial list of the diseases causing cor pulmonale include: COPD, AIDS, primary pulmonary hypertension, and chronic pulmonary emboli.

The "sine qua non" of cor pulmonale is pulmonary artery hypertension, with a pulmonary artery pressure at rest of greater than 20 mm Hg. The two most common factors leading to increase pulmonary artery pressure are: 1. alveolar hypoxia which is by far the most common, at least in COPD, kyphoscoliosis, and the obesity–hypoventilation syndrome, and 2. structural changes in the pulmonary vascular bed (pulmonary vascular remodeling).

The gold standard for diagnosing cor pulmonale is the direct measurement of pressures in the right ventricle and pulmonary artery but for many patients the procedure is fraught with risk. Ultrasound evaluation has been used but is just not as accurate. Magnetic Resonance Imaging (MRI) produces the best images of the right ventricle and is likely the best non-invasive tool available to study cor pulmonale. In COPD patients there is a good correlation between right ventricular volume measured by MRI and the pulmonary artery pressure.

Patients with cor pulmonale present with fatigue, dyspnea, cough and occasionally chest pain due to a form of angina related to right ventricular strain. The hallmark clinical sign of cor pulmonale is the presence of pedal edema. Other findings include neck vein distention, liver enlargement, ascites (fluid in the peritoneal space) and pleural effusions.

The acute treatment of right heart failure is the use of diuretics and oxygen. The long-term treatment of cor pulmonale is oxygen therapy for patients who are hypoxic as well as vasodilators for patients with type 1 PAH. The underlying pulmonary condition causing the cor pulmonale must be addressed.

The prognosis of cor pulmonale is determined by the underlying cause of the disorder.

IMPORTANT CONCEPTS TO REMEMBER FROM THIS LECTURE

1. Poiseuille's Law relates:
   The flow rate in a tube to the pressure gradient and resistance. The greater the pressure gradient the greater the flow; the greater the resistance the slower the flow

2. Starling's law relates:
   The net flow of fluids in and out of a vessel is due to the difference between the colloid osmotic pressure in the vessel and interstitium and the difference in pressure inside the vessel which pushes out and the pressure outside the vessel which pushes in.

3. The driving pressure in the pulmonary system is:
   One tenth that in the systemic system.

4. Cor Pulmonale is seen with
   COPD, AIDS, primary pulmonary hypertension, and chronic pulmonary emboli

Lecture Seven

The Upper Airway

The Nose and Nasopharynx

The upper airway is a huge chamber that includes the nose and nasopharynx, the mouth and oral pharynx, as well as the larynx or hypopharynx. Each part of the upper airway has its own anatomy and each part has its own function.

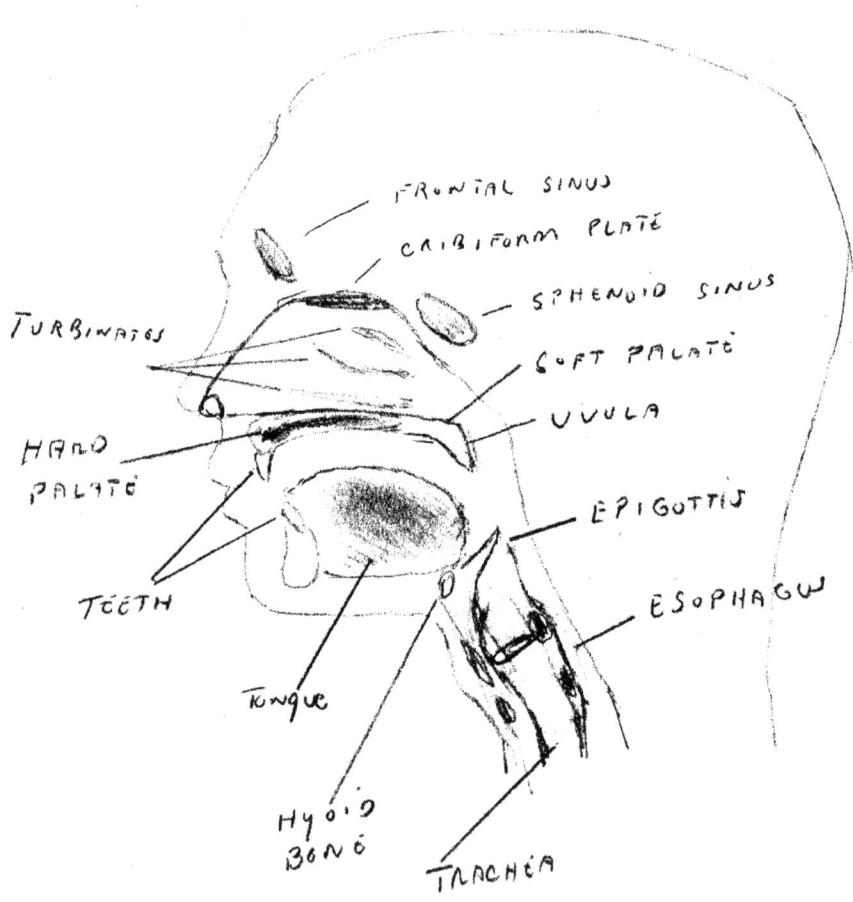

Side view of the pharynx showing the nasal cavity with its three turbinates and two of its four sinuses, the oral pharynx with the tongue and uvula, and the hypopharynx with the epiglottis and posterior esophagus.

The nose is most often taken for granted, except, of course, by plastic surgeons, whose livelihood depends upon our dislike of our own anatomy. In reality, it is truly an incredible work of art.

The anterior portion of the nose functions as a brush to cleanse the air that we breathe of contaminants both large and small. The little hairs called vibrissae latch onto the large particles while the mucous that coats the nasal passage binds noxious gases. In addition, the mucosa functions as a counter-current humidifier and heater. When we breathe out we warm and humidify the nasal lining. When we breathe in the nasal lining transfers the warmth and moisture to the incoming air. Cold air can cause asthma. This countercurrent mechanism helps prevent it. Irritating the vibrissae of a dog with a predisposition to asthma will provoke wheezing in the creature suggesting a neural connection between the nasal mucosa and the vagal nerves to the lungs.

The epithelial lining of the anterior part of the nose is stratified squamous epithelium similar to our skin while the posterior part, the nasopharynx, is lined by pseudostratified ciliated columnar epithelium which is the same type of epithelium that we have in our trachea and large airways. But why should this be the case? Why should the nasopharynx share the same type of epithelium with the trachea? The back of the mouth, called the oropharynx, doesn't. Neither does the larynx.

Four sinuses arise from the nasopharynx: the frontal sinuses, located above the eyes, the maxillary sinuses, located in the cheek bones, the ethmoid sinuses located on the sides of the nose and sphenoid sinuses at the very back of the nasopharynx. The function of the sinuses is somewhat obscure. Perhaps, because they are hollow, they lower the weight of the skull and allow us to stand tall. They also produce the mucous which lines our nasal cavity. But they can become infected causing sinusitis.

Lastly the Eustachian Tube or Auditory Tube arises along the sides of the posterior nasopharynx and connects the nose to the middle ear. The tube keeps the pressure in the middle ear near the atmospheric pressure and also drains secretions and debris from the middle ear. The tube is normally closed but when we yawn or swallow it opens briefly equalizing the pressure between the nose and middle ear. Occasionally we hear or feel a popping when this happens. If the channel becomes blocked due to severe allergic rhinitis or a viral infection, an infection in the middle ear can result, which is called *Otitis Media*.

For some of us, the most important function of the nose is smell. At the very top of the nose is a plate, the olfactory plate, which separates the nose from the brain directly above it. The plate is pierced by millions of tiny holes. A tiny nerve ending fills each little hole. The nerve endings unite above the nose and form the Olfactory Nerve or Cranial Nerve 1 which travels directly to the brain. The nerve endings are extremely sensitive and can interpret thousands of different types of smell. Even more important, if we lose the sense of smell, perhaps due to a head injury or because of chronic allergic symptoms, we partially lose our ability to taste. Taste and smell go together like hand and finger.

The Mouth and Oral Pharynx

The oral pharynx consists of an anterior portion called the vestibule as well as the posterior oral pharynx. The mouth is important in speech, taste, and swallowing.

The top of the mouth is formed by the palate which separates the mouth from the nose. The anterior portion is made up of a bony plate and is called the *hard palate*; the posterior portion is composed of soft tissues and is called the *soft palate*. There is a flap of tissue dripping down from the distal end of the soft palate which is called the *Uvula*. The word Uvula comes from a Latin work meaning a "bundle of grapes." If you touch your uvula you will gag! But then, why do we have a Uvula at all? Some patients with sleep apnea are treated by removing the soft tissue at the back of the mouth, making the opening from the mouth to the larynx larger and firmer. The surgery is called an *uvulopalatopharyngoplasty* (UPPP). Afterwards many of the patients find they have a more nasal voice and more nasal reflux when they drink liquids.

It is likely that the Uvula is an accessory organ of speech, important in the French and certain Arabic languages. It also helps prevent food from entering the nose when we swallow. Some researchers suggest that it is also immunologically important because it contains an area of macrophages and T cell lymphocytes just below its epithelium. Another researcher suggested that a long uvula might cause cough by irritating the upper airway!

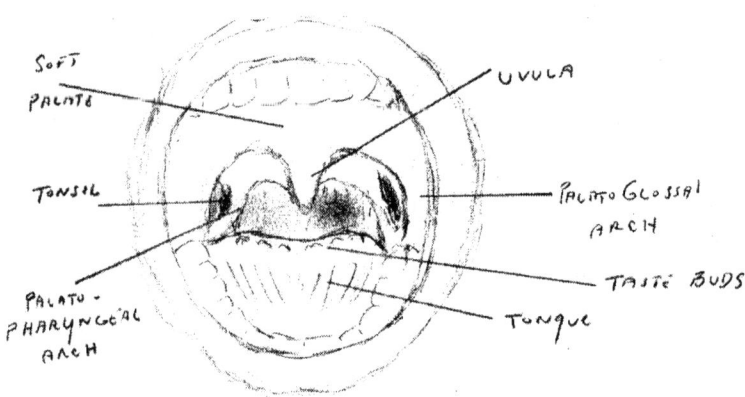

The oral pharynx from the dentist's view. The two arches surround the tonsils. On the back of the tongue is a row of mounds which are the large taste bloods.

The back of the mouth is the oral pharynx which is in direct communication with the nasopharynx above and hypopharynx or laryngopharynx below. On both sides of the oral pharynx are two pillars, the anterior palatoglossal and posterior palatopharyngeal pillars, between which lie the tonsils. Most importantly, the internal carotid arteries, which supply blood to our brain, are located directly behind the tonsils.

The oral cavity and oral pharynx are both lined by squamous epithelium.

The base of the mouth is the tongue, a very large muscle which inserts on the hyoid bone, which is actually a cartilage and not a bone at all. It is the large U like structure you can readily feel about two inches back of your chin where your chin joins your neck.

Certainly, the most important function of our mouth is taste. Taste is a function of the row of taste buds found traversing the top of the tongue posteriorly. They look like a V-shaped, transverse row of tiny tumors.

Taste is affected by our sense of smell, the texture of the food, and whether the food causes pain. Pepper doesn't excite the taste receptors; rather it excites the pain receptors. The primary sensations of taste are: sour, salty, sweet, bitter, and "Umami". Sourness is a response to acids in our food. Salty taste is a response to the concentration of sodium in the food. Bitter taste is the most sensitive taste and is a response to long chained, nitrogen containing alkaloids such as caffeine, strychnine, and nicotine. "Umami" is a Japanese word that means "delicious". This sensation is due to L-glutamate present in meat extracts and aged cheese.

Hypopharynx or Laryngopharynx

For most of us and even, I'm sure, for many Respiratory Therapy students, the hypopharynx ranks right up there with the appendix and gallbladder. But for me, the hypopharynx is one of the four most important organs in the body and the only one that is important in two entirely separate bodily functions. How could I possibly rate the hypopharynx up there with the brain, heart, and lungs? The student will correctly point out that diseases of the hypopharynx don't even rank in the top twenty causes of death.

But diseases of the hypopharynx do cause extensive disease and death. Remember the larynx is important not only in breathing but also in swallowing. Without a functioning larynx swallowing becomes impossible. If you are unable to swallow food because it lodges in the esophagus you quickly become malnourished. If, on the other hand, every time you sip water or eat a bit of food you choke or aspirate, you soon stop eating and you become emaciated. Severe weight loss impairs your immune system which stops functioning and you get an infection like pneumonia and you die. Pneumonia certainly ranks among the top ten causes of death in America.

Structurally, the hypopharynx divides the pharynx into two tubes, an anterior, round to slightly oval tube which is buttressed on the front and both sides by cartilage while the posterior wall abuts on a soft tube, the esophagus, which most of the time, is flattened in its anterior-to posterior dimension, and which is made up entirely of soft tissue.

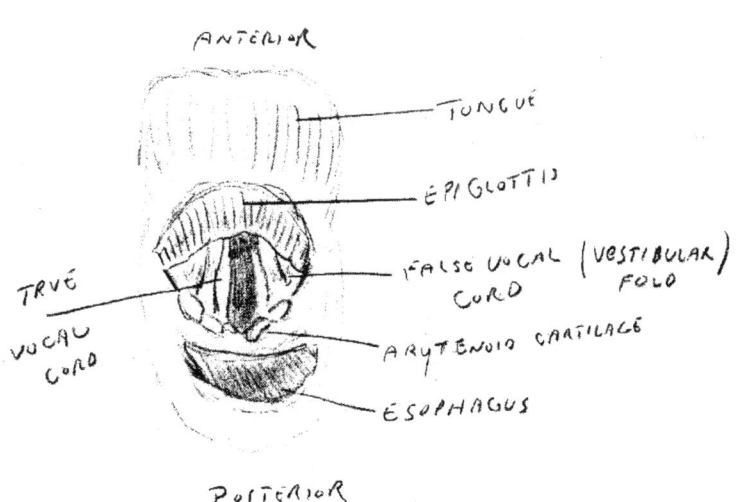

Looking down at the hypopharynx from above. The tongue is at the top. Below the tongue is the epiglottis and then the glottis composed of the vocal cords. The vocal cords attach to the thyroid cartilage anteriorly and the arytenoid cartilages posteriorly. Behind the larynx is the opening into the esophagus which is closed.

The anterior tube is the larynx and the posterior tube the esophagus. The larynx tends to maintain its shape whereas the esophagus is collapsed except when we eat or drink something.

The larynx is composed of nine cartilages. At the top, anteriorly, is the hyoid bone, actually a cartilage, which on its superior surface is attached to the base of the tongue and on its inferior surface to the muscles of the larynx. The hyoid bone is easily palpable. It is the U shaped, bow-like cartilage that you feel at the angle where your chin diverges anteriorly from your neck.

The epiglottis arises immediately below and posterior to the hyoid bone. It is pointed over the top of the larynx. The epiglottis has long been thought to be the protector of the airway. When we swallow the epiglottis closes over the larynx keeping food and water out of our airway. But the true protector of our airway is the pair of vocal cords which clamp tight when we swallow. When we swallow the larynx is pulled upwards and the epiglottis becomes a "cap" which deflects the food and liquid into the esophagus.

Below the epiglottis is the largest cartilage of the larynx, the thyroid cartilage. It is called the thyroid cartilage because the thyroid gland is located immediately in front of and to the sides of the cartilage. The thyroid cartilage forms the "Adam's Apple". The thyroid cartilage is connected by a membrane to the hyoid bone above it. At the top of the cartilage anteriorly, in the very center, is the thyroid notch.

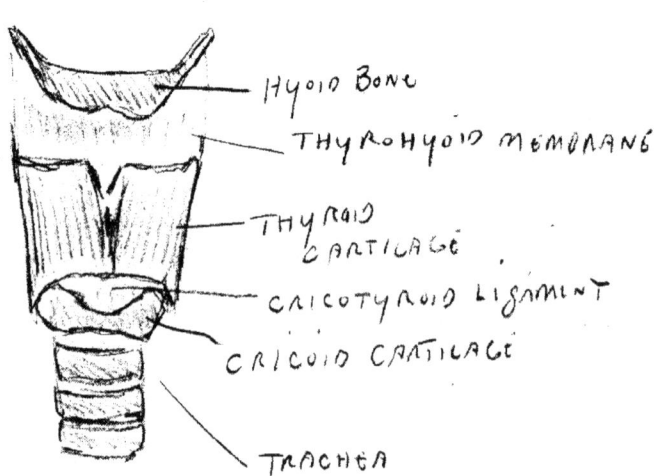

Anterior View of the Larynx

There is a pair of arytenoid cartilages arising along the posterior wall of the larynx directly across from the back of the thyroid cartilage. The vocal cords attach to these small cartilages as do several muscles. The vocal cords attach anteriorly to the back of the thyroid cartilage.

The vocal cords are made up of folds of membranous tissue with a few strands of muscle. They are pearly white in color, and most importantly, form the narrowest part of the air passage which is called the *glottis*. Male vocal cords are longer and thicker and for that reason most men have a lower pitched voice. The superior surface of the vocal cords is lined by stratified squamous epithelium similar to the oropharynx while the inferior surface is lined by pseudostratified ciliated columnar epithelium which, of course, is the main epithelium of the trachea and major bronchi.

The lowest cartilage of the larynx is the cricoid cartilage which forms a ring around the lower margin of the structure. Anteriorly, between the thyroid and cricoid cartilage is a membranous structure, the cricothyroid membrane which is the site used for emergency tracheotomies.

<u>The trachea begins immediately below the cricoid cartilage</u>.

The larynx is also a very muscular organ with muscles needed not only for phonation but also for elevating and closing off the larynx during swallowing and the Valsalva maneuver. The larynx is innervated by the Vagus Nerve (10th cranial nerve) for sensation and the Glossopharyngeal Nerve (9th cranial nerve) for muscular activity.

During quiet inhalation, the vocal cords spread apart and widen the glottis, while during exhalation they close slightly, always remaining a little open. But during the Valsalva maneuver as well as at the onset of a cough, the larynx closes tightly. There is adduction of the laryngeal walls (the walls of the larynx squeeze together), including both the true and false vocal cords. The glottis is tightly sealed. During a cough the muscles of the abdomen and chest tighten, building pressure in the thorax. When the glottis opens, there is an extremely forceful flow of air.

Speech originates in the motor cortex. The brain decides what it is going to say and how it will say it. The cortex then communicates with Broca's Area, the lowest part of the motor cortex, which organizes the neural output. The signal passes to the brainstem, the most primitive part of our brain. The brainstem controls our breathing, our larynx and vocal cords while we speak as well as the tongue and other parts of the mouth which shape or articulate the sound. The brain then interprets the results and makes fine adjustments.

Swallowing is even more complex. In the first step food is squeezed into the posterior oral pharynx by the pressure of the tongue upwards and the palate backwards. The soft palate is pulled upwards to close off the nasopharynx. The folds of the larynx are pulled medially, channeling the food into the esophagus. The vocal cords close off the glottis completely. Then the larynx is pulled upwards enlarging the opening of the esophagus as the epiglottis caps the larynx. Then the entire muscular wall of the pharynx contracts forcing the bolus of food into the esophagus.

The swallowing center is found in areas in the medulla and lower pons portions of the brainstem and is responsible for coordinating the pharyngeal phase of swallowing. A disease of the brainstem will impair swallowing resulting in aspiration. Cranial nerves 5, 9, 10, and 12 are all involved. The swallowing center turns off the respiratory center during the swallowing maneuver and breathing ceases.

Common Disorders of the Upper Airways.

The most common disorder of the nasopharynx is, of course, the "common cold". It is a self-limited, viral illness, usually lasting a few days and characterized by a runny nose with nasal stuffiness. While the patient feels terrible he or she doesn't have a cough or fever. By the time the patient succeeds in getting an appointment with his or her doctor, the illness is almost over.

"Sinusitis" on the other hand is often a very severe illness. It is defined as an "inflammation" of the sinuses and it is the most common cause of a visit to the doctor. Thirty million Americans get sinusitis every year. The classic symptoms are purulent nasal drainage, facial pain (usually over the check bones), and nasal obstruction. But sinusitis involving the sphenoid or ethmoid sinuses can present with pain at the top of the head or even the back of the head. The main physical finding is tenderness over the maxillary sinuses, which are the most common sinuses involved in the illness. Pus might be seen in the anterior nares or dripping into the oral pharynx. In patients who have allergic rhinitis along with their sinus infection, nasal polyps may be seen.

The cause of acute sinusitis is usually a viral infection. The most common bacterial sinus infections are due to the Pneumococcus, Hemophilus, and Moraxella bacteria. Chronic sinusitis is usually **not** an infectious disease.

The diagnosis is often made clinically, but radiographic findings are classic. There is thickening of the wall of the sinuses and an air-fluid level present.

The treatment involves sinus irrigation, an intranasal steroid spray and usually an antibiotic. Surgery may be required in the treatment of chronic sinusitis.

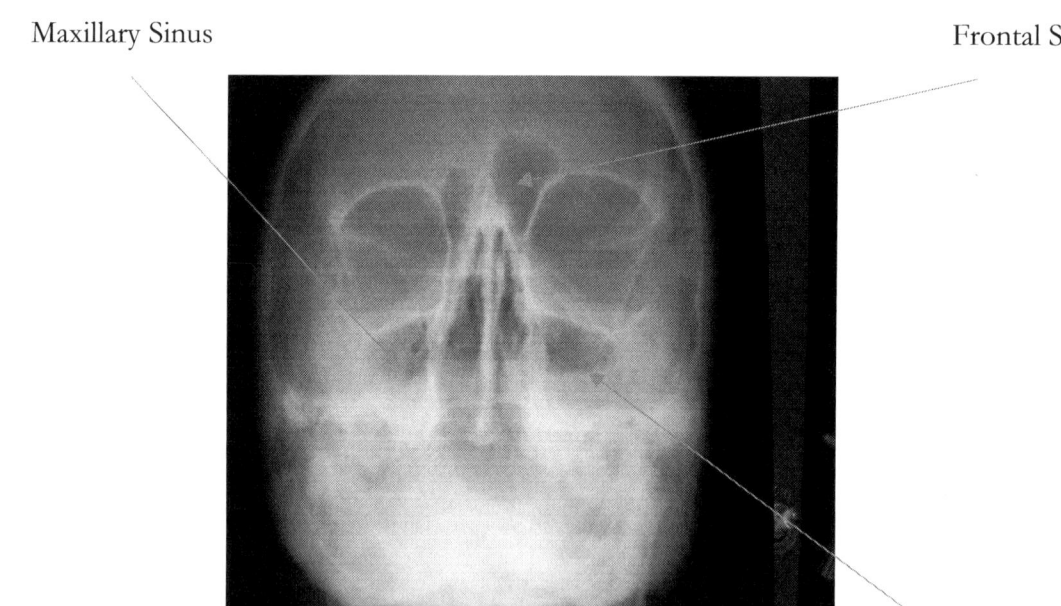

Maxillary Sinus

Frontal Sinus

Air fluid level

Pharyngitis or "sore throat" is most often due to a viral infection. But during winter about 20% of the general population grows Pneumococcal bacterium on throat culture.

Diphtheria is a very rare throat infection. It is caused by the bacterium Corynebacterium diphtheria. In the last forty years the disease has become quite rare in the developed world but recently has recurred in Yemen. Before 1980 there were a million cases a year world-wide but in recent years, till the outbreak in war-torn Yemen there have only been about 4-5000 cases a year. It generally affects children and has a 10% mortality. The illness is characterized by a severe pharyngitis. The throat is covered by a thick, grey, membranous tissue which can block the airway. Complications include inflammation of the heart, nerves and kidneys, as well as a bleeding disorder due to thrombocytopenia (low platelets). The disease is preventable with a vaccine.

Thrush is a common cause of a sore throat in infants. The pharynx, tongue, and even the inner surface of the cheek is covered by myriads of tiny creamy white patches. The infection is due to the fungus Candida albicans. There are two causes in adults. The first is the use of orally-inhaled steroids in a patient with asthma. The second occurs in immunologically compromised people such as patients suffering from AIDS or the Adult Immuno-Deficiency Syndrome.

Epiglottitis is inflammation of the epiglottis and is most often caused by the bacterium Hemophilus influenzae, Type B. It affects infants and causes swelling of the epiglottis. This is a true medical emergency. Intubation or even a tracheostomy may be required to maintain the infant's airway but must be done in a controlled environment. Do not examine or manipulate the epiglottis in an uncontrolled situation if you suspect the patient has epiglottitis.

Acute Laryngospasm may follow extubation, even if the patient has been intubated for a short time. The diagnosis is established clinically by the presence of stridor, which is a high-pitched monophonic wheeze audible at the mouth. The treatment is re-intubation and then a short course of steroid prior to a second go at extubation.

Rheumatoid arthritis, an autoimmune disorder, which causes diffuse arthritis of the hands and other joints, may also cause "arthritis" of the arytenoid cartilages which function as true joints just like the joints in the fingers. The patient may present with hoarseness, total loss of his or her voice or even severe shortness of breath.

Vocal Cord Dysfunction is another disorder of the larynx. This disorder mimics asthma. The patient has the sudden onset of wheezing and shortness of breath which is unresponsive to Beta adrenergic agents and steroids but which resolves as quickly as it began when the patient is intubated. The diagnosis is made by directly observing the vocal cords during an attack. The treatment is relaxation therapy. A second less common though no less severe disorder is Vocal Cord Spasm. This is a neurological disorder which causes persistent hoarseness. It is due to disease of the same part of the brain that causes Parkinson's disease. The treatment is with Botox injections of the vocal cords to prevent the spasm.

The last disorder of the hypopharynx is the most severe. This is chronic aspiration. Even college students aspirate on a daily basis. As we age the aspiration becomes more frequent. Pneumonia is the direct result of aspiration. The swallowing center is an autonomic nerve center located in the brainstem. Many patients develop brainstem disease due to small strokes, atherosclerosis, or degenerative diseases such as ALS (Amyotrophic Lateral Sclerosis) known as Lou Gehrig's disease if you're my age or Stephen Hawking's disease if you're a college student. The treatment is supportive. Even a tracheostomy is of little value.

IMPORTANT CONCEPTS TO REMEMBER FROM THIS LECTURE

1. Where is pseudostratified ciliated columnar epithelium found?

>   Posterior nasopharynx, trachea and large airways.

2. The tonsils are found in a curtain like structure in the lateral posterior oral pharynx. The tonsils are associated in this location with:

>   The internal carotid arteries.

3. The cricoid cartilage is located directly above:

>   The trachea.

4. The Cricothyroid Ligament is:

>   Located between the thyroid and cricoid cartilages and is often used for percutaneous emergency tracheostomy.

Lecture Eight

The Chest Wall

The easiest way to approach the chest wall is to study it in layers. The outermost layer is, of course, the skin and all its appendages. Below that the bony cage protects the vital organs of the thorax. Muscles connect the bony structures and allow us to breathe. Immediately inside the bony cage lies the two layered pleural lining of the lungs.

Skin

Our outer layer, the skin, might at first seem unimportant. However, it has several important functions. The skin protects us against pathogens. Sweat has unique antibacterial properties. It is hypotonic and composed mostly of water, with only a little salt. It also has antibodies, and a chemical called dermicidin, which is an antimicrobial peptide. (Peptides are small proteins.) Antimicrobial peptides turn out to be one of the primary mechanisms used by the skin for immune defense. These antimicrobial peptides have shown broad antibacterial activity against not only gram-positive and gram-negative bacteria but even some fungi and viruses.

The skin provides insulation and prevents dehydration and aids in temperature regulation. Most importantly, it produces Vitamin D which helps the body absorb Calcium from the gut. Vitamin D is important not only in preventing a bone disease called rickets in children and osteomalacia in adults but it plays a role in glucose regulation and in the workings of the immune system.

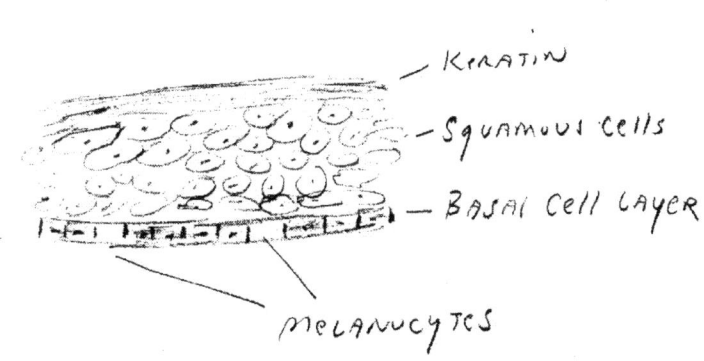

The Epidermis is the top layer of the skin. Skin is made up of stacked layers of squamous cells covered by keratin which is a fibrous protein. The melanocytes are found in the basal layer.

The skin consists of three layers: the epidermis, the dermis, and the subcutaneous layer. The epidermis is the outer layer. It is made up of stratified squamous cells as well as the melanocytes which give us our skin color. The dermis is largely connective tissue but it houses the sweat cells, nerves, hair follicles, and blood vessels. The lowest level is the subcutaneous tissue composed of fat and connective tissue.

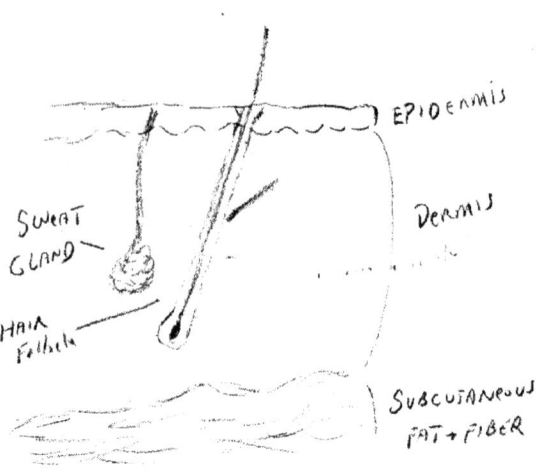

The skin consists of three levels: 1. the epidermis, 2. the dermis which contains not only the sweat glands and hair follicles but also the nerves, vascular structure and lymphatics, and 3. the subcutaneous layer which is made up of fat and fiber.

The skin is up to 14 mm (nearly 1 and ½ centimeters) thick over the back but only a half millimeter thick around the eye.

There are many skin disorders which can affect the chest wall but the two most important are "shingles" and melanomas.

"Shingles" is due to infection with the chicken pox virus. The primary infection with the Varicella-Zoster virus generally occurs during childhood. The virus is extremely contagious. It causes a generalized skin rash which lasts a few days. The rash is extremely itchy with red blisters. It begins over the face and thorax and then spreads to the rest of the body. It can also cause pneumonia, especially if the infection occurs during the late teens, and encephalitis, which is an infection of the brain tissue. In 2013 there were over 140,000,000 cases of chicken pox with 6000 deaths worldwide.

The virus then enters the nervous system and lies dormant. As the patient ages his or her immune system begins to fail, perhaps due to cancer, diabetes or just growing old. When it does the virus migrates from spinal cord, where it has bided its time, out the nerves to the skin where it causes a very painful and often deforming rash called "Shingles". The rash generally lasts about 2 months but the pain, a type of neuropathy or "nerve pain", can last for many months or even years. The rash is red and blistery and is located along a *dermatome*. Thus if the rash involves the fifth thoracic nerves on the right, the rash will extend from the mid-back around the chest wall to the nipples only the right side. The rash is almost always unilateral and almost always in a linear pattern.

Sometimes, however the patient can have pain without the rash ever occurring, making the diagnosis very difficult to establish.

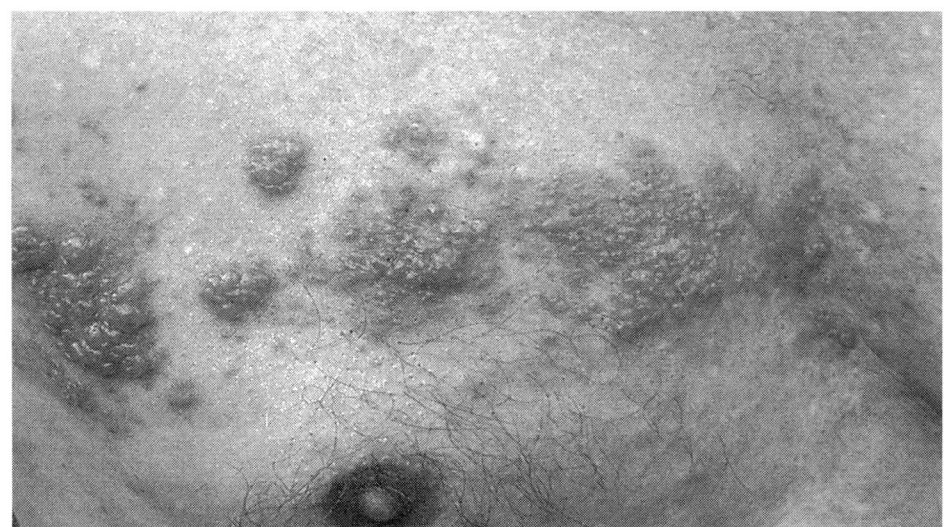

The characteristic blisters of Herpes Zoster or Shingles.

Getting the chicken pox vaccine as a child should prevent getting "Shingles" as an adult. There are now two "shingles" vaccines. The first, Zostavax is simply a very large dose of the children's chicken pox vaccine. It is about 70% effective. Since it is a live virus vaccine precautions must be taken to avoid spreading chicken pox to unvaccinated children and adults. The newest vaccine, Shingrix, requires two shots be given two to six months apart, but it is non-living and thus can't be transmitted, and it is more than 90% effective.

A *Melanoma* is a cancer of the skin which arises from the melanocytes. It generally appears as a small, irregular, red to black elevated lesion on the skin. What most of us don't realize is that a Melanoma can occur anywhere on the body not just where the sun shines. The youngest patient I've seen with a lung cancer was a 27 year old woman with a left lung mass which turned out to be a melanoma.

Melanomas appear to be immunologic tumors. Every time you get a sunburn anywhere on your skin, your risk of getting a melanoma doubles and the cancer can occur anywhere on, or in, your body.

Bony Thorax and Musculature

The bony thorax consists of the vertebral column, the sternum, and ribs that span the sternum and backbone.

The sternum forms the anterior border of the chest wall and is composed of three parts: the manubrium, the body of the sternum, and the xiphoid process. The articulation between the manubrium and the body of the sternum is an easily palpable transverse ridge near the top of the sternum. It is called the Angle of Louis. The trachea bifurcates into the right and left bronchus directly behind the sternum at this level. Directly behind the sternal notch is the trachea itself. The trachea should always be in the mid line. The lowest part of the sternum is the xiphoid process.

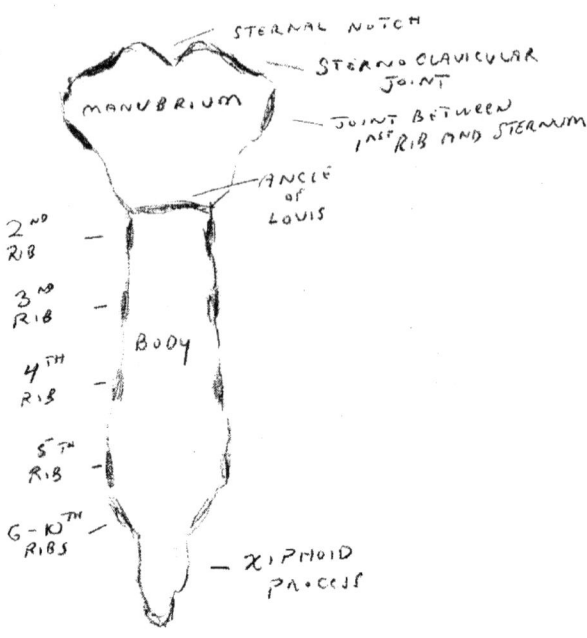

The sternum consists of three parts, the manubrium, the body, and the tiny xiphoid process

The rib cage forms the lateral boundary of the thorax. The ribs are attached to the vertebral column posteriorly and most are attached, one way or another, to the sternum anteriorly.

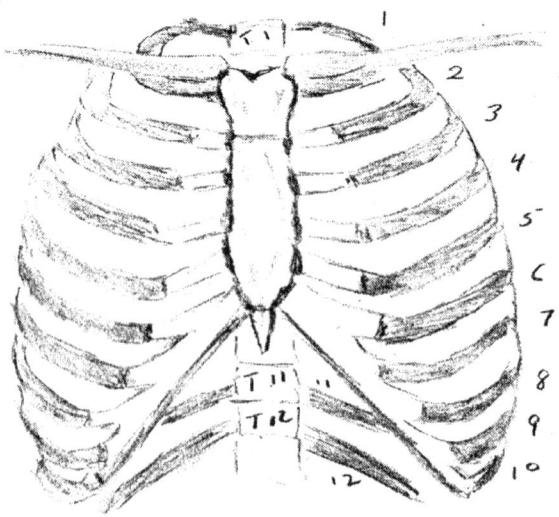

The rib cage showing the sternum and ribs. The white areas between the gray ribs and the sternum are the cartilaginous joints.

The backbone or thoracic vertebra forms the posterior border of the thorax. The junction between the vertebral column and the ribs is a joint, just like the joints in our fingers, hips, and knees.

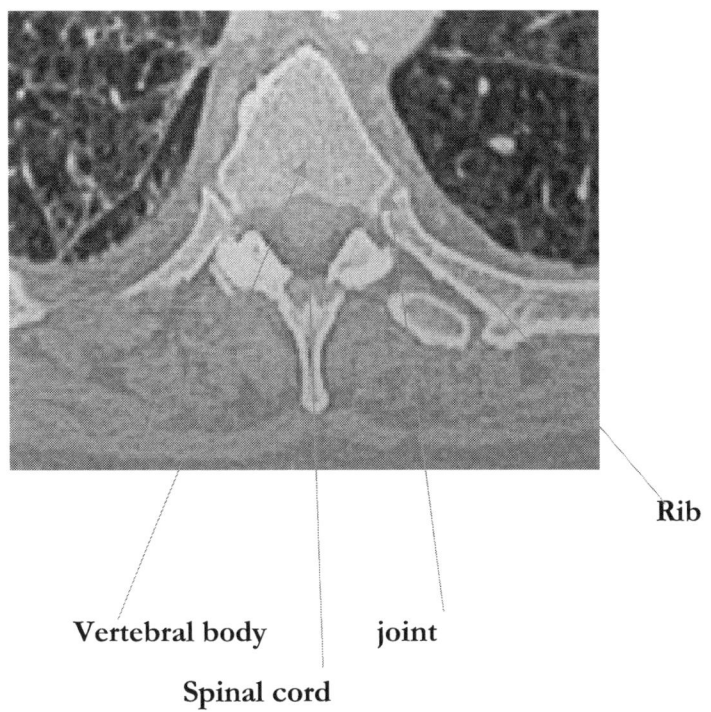

Vertebral body   **joint**   **Rib**

Spinal cord

The ribs are a little more complex. The first seven ribs attach directly to the sternum and are called the *True Ribs*. The bony ribs and the bony sternum are separated by a cartilaginous joint and thus can move independently. The eighth through tenth ribs insert into the seventh ribs and are called the *False Ribs* while the last two ribs are very short and cover just the back part of the thorax. They are referred to as the *Floating Ribs*.

The spaces between the ribs are called the intercostal spaces. The space between the 2nd and 3rd ribs is the 2nd intercostal space. There is a small groove on the **inferior** surface of the rib in which the intercostal nerve, artery, and vein are found. The external intercostal muscles are located between the ribs and are adjacent to the subcutaneous tissue. The external intercostal muscles overlie the internal intercostal muscles which are adjacent to the parietal pleura.

There are several disorders which can affect the chest wall. These include congenital abnormalities including *funnel chest* and *pigeon breast*. Of the two, Funnel Chest has more serious consequences. The chest wall curves inward at the sternum. The heart is forced into the left hemithorax compressing the lung and causing a restriction of lung volume. Pigeon breast is just the opposite, the sternum is thrust forward. Unlike funnel chest there is no restriction of lung volumes. However, pigeon breast is associated with cyanotic heart disorders.

Osteomyelitis, which is an infection of the bone, is very uncommon but when it occurs is most often due to Staphylococcus aureus or pseudomonas infections. Tuberculosis of the ribs or sternum is usually due to spread from a lung infection. Pott's disease is a tuberculosis infection of the spine, usually starting in the cartilaginous joint between the spine and the rib. It is one of the oldest diseases of mankind, having been identified in the skeletal remains of people who lived in the Iron Age in Europe as well as in mummies from ancient Egypt.

Vitamin D deficiency is the most common disease of the bony thorax. In children it causes Rickets, in adults it cause osteomalacia. Rickets and Osteomalacia are exactly the same even though they have different names. Both conditions are due to calcium deficiency in the bones causing "soft bones". They are generally due to malnutrition. Vitamin D is required for the absorption of calcium by the gut. No vitamin D means no calcium in the bones. The bones bend and break easily. The child with Rickets is bow-legged and has a history of frequent fractures. Typically, there is a Rachitic Rosary characterized by bony lumps or beads outlining the costochondral junctions.

Muscles

The major muscle of breathing is the diaphragm. This is the large muscle which separates the abdomen from the chest. It is thick, flat, and dome-shaped. There are, in reality, two hemidiaphragms, one for each thorax, which are fused together by a central tendon. The edges of the large muscle attach in the back to the vertebral column, along the sides to the lower rib cage, and anteriorly to the xiphoid process. There are three large openings of the diaphragm, one for the aorta, one for the vena cava, and one for the esophagus.

The diaphragm is innervated by the *phrenic nerves* which originate from the 3rd, 4th, and 5th cervical nerves. The phrenic nerve is motor only. There are no sensory fibers. But even though it doesn't have sensory fibers, irritation of the diaphragm, such as by an infected gallbladder, can cause pain, but not pain in the diaphragm, rather pain in the shoulder area. This is called referred pain and is due to the fact that signals travel up the phrenic nerve back to the cervical spine and then out the 3rd, 4th, and 5th cervical nerves to the shoulder area which they also innervate. Thus gallbladder pain can be felt in the right shoulder and pain from a pulmonary infarct in the lung directly above the dome of the left hemidiaphragm can be felt in the left shoulder.

The diaphragm and external intercostal muscles are the muscles of quiet inspiration or inhalation. In men, only the diaphragm may be involved in quiet inspiration. When the diaphragm contracts it is pulled downward expanding the thorax. When the external intercostal muscles contract they pull the thorax upwards and outwards. Both these effects results in a fall in intrathoracic pressure. When the intrathoracic pressure is less than the pressure at the mouth, air flows into the lungs.

No muscle activity at all is required for quiet exhalation because of the elastic properties of the chest wall and lungs.

When forceful inspiration is necessary, like when we are running, several other muscles can be called upon to aid inspiration including the Scalene and Sternocleidomastoid muscles of the neck, the Pectoralis Major muscle of the anterior chest wall, and the large Trapezius Muscle of the upper back. All these muscles have other functions such as turning the head, bending the head, hugging or shrugging, but by fixating their bony insertions in the spine and shoulder, they can aid inspiration.

There are two groups of muscles that can be called upon to increase the force of exhalation. The first group is the intrinsic intercostal muscles which narrow the chest wall by pulling the ribs downward and inward, just the opposite of the extrinsic intercostal muscles. The second group is the collection of large abdominal muscles which, when they contract, push the diaphragm up into the chest. These include the Rectus abdominis muscles, External abdominis oblique muscles, internal abdominis oblique muscles and the transversus abdominis muscles.

The Pleura and Pleural Space

The pleura lies just under the ribs and is made up of two layers. The outer layer is called the *parietal pleura*. It is affixed to the inner surface of the ribs and intercostal spaces, to the top (thoracic side) of the diaphragm, and to the mediastinum. The inner layer is called the *visceral pleura*. It directly overlays and adheres to the lung itself. Between the two layers is the *pleural space*. Normally, the pleural space contains less than ten cc of a serous fluid. It is called "serous" because it is watery substance which has only a few white cells and a very low protein content. The fluid serves as a lubricant allowing the lungs to move freely in the chest cavity. The parietal pleura manufactures about 1.5 cc a day of pleural fluid. The fluid is drained by lymphatics found in the parietal pleura which can remove up to 500 cc a day.

Most importantly, only the parietal pleura has sensory fibers. The visceral pleura has **no** nerve fibers!

The pleural space always has a negative pressure. At rest, the chest wall tends to pull out while the lungs, like an inflated balloon, tend to collapse. If a knife is imbedded in the chest creating a hole, the lungs will collapse and the chest wall will expand. In the closed thorax, the negative pleural pressure creates a constant tug on the lungs helping to keep them open and also tends to draw fluid into the space which must be removed by the lymphatics. But the negative pressure, which is normally about -5 cm. at the base of the lungs is less than a third of what would be needed to suck air out of the capillaries underlying the parietal pleura.

Diseases of the Pleural Space

Diseases of the pleural space include a *pneumothorax* in which the pleural space fills with air and a pleural effusion in which a liquid of some type fills part of the pleural space.

A pneumothorax is often due to direct chest wall trauma such as when a fractured rib pierces the lung and air from the lung escapes into the pleural space. Usually the hole between the lung and the pleural space is open only during inspiration when the pleural pressure is low so that more and more air become trapped outside the lung with each breath. The expanding air pushes the lung towards the other hemithorax and the circulation becomes compromised. This is called a tension pneumothorax and requires immediate action.

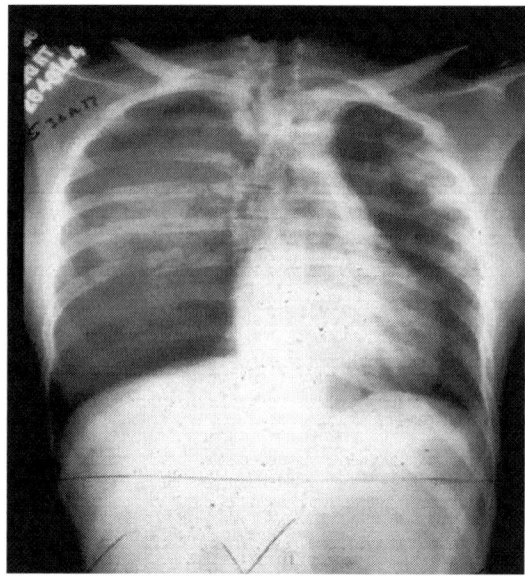

The CXR shows a moderate sized right pneumothorax. The clues are that the lung appears whiter because when it collapses it is denser. There is a well-defined demarcation between the whitish lung and the air-filled pneumothorax. This is a tension pneumothorax because the heart is shifted away from the pneumothorax. Lastly there are numerous black streaks suggesting air in the mediastinum. The CXR is that of a motorcyclist.

Pleural effusions are collections of fluid in the pleural space between the visceral and parietal pleura. They are fairly common. There are two types: transudates and exudates.

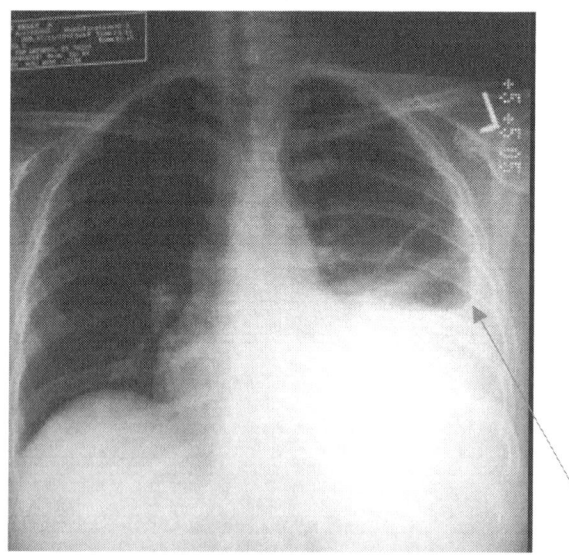

Meniscus sign

The CXR shows a large left pleural effusion with a pronounced meniscus sign. The fluid seems to climb up the wall of the thorax.

Transudates are non-inflammatory. There are few cells and the fluid has a low protein content. The pleura is not directly involved in their creation. Rather transudates are generally caused by decreased drainage of fluid by the lymphatic system. Increased pressure in the blood vessels will cause the lymphatic drainage system to fail by blocking the thoracic duct. The most common cause is congestive heart failure. In addition, if the lymphatic drainage system is blocked by a tumor, most often a breast cancer, pleural fluid will build up.

Another cause of a transudate is cirrhosis of the liver. Cirrhosis causes ascites which is the accumulation of fluid in the abdomen. The increased pressure in the abdomen can force open small pores in the diaphragm and allow fluid to enter the chest.

Exudates are due to diseases that involve the pleural space directly. Exudates usually are quite cellular and have a high protein content. Cancers, especially lung and breast cancer, and infections such as tuberculosis, can involve the pleural space and cause an exudate.

An *empyema* is when the pleural space becomes filled with pus usually from a bacterial infection. A *hemothorax* is when the pleural space is filled with blood, usually after trauma such as a broken rib or other form of penetrating injury to the chest wall.

The pleural effusion will be seen on the chest x-ray if it is over 300 cc. The costophrenic angle, which normally looks like a check mark, will be absent or blunted. The hallmark finding is the *meniscus* sign. The fluid, instead of being a flat line as in an air-fluid level, appears to creep up the side of the chest wall. It is due to the attraction of the water molecule for the pleural lining.

The heart should be pushed away from the side of the effusion. If is not, look for an associated atelectasis of the lung.

The pleural fluid, if large enough, will compress the underlying lung causing atelectasis resulting in an area of low ventilation and hypoxemia. In addition, if the effusion is very large it will push the heart into the contralateral hemithorax obstructing venous return. It may even compress the large veins. Either effect will cause the cardiac output to fall.

The first step in evaluating a collection of pleural fluid is to get a sample of the fluid by doing a *thoracentesis*. Simply put, a thoracentesis involves putting a needle directly into the pleural space and either collecting a sample of the fluid or draining the fluid completely. Most importantly, because the intercostal arteries, veins and nerves are located on the inferior surface of the rib, the needle must be inserted above the rib and not below it.

The Lungs

When you open the thorax, the lung looks like a mushroom. It is a large, soft, air-filled bulbous structure supported by a stalk. You can actually grab the stalk in your hands and wave the lung about. The stalk is called the *hilum*. The hilum contains the main stem bronchi, the pulmonary artery and vein, the large lymph channels and lymph nodes, as well as the sympathetic and parasympathetic nerves which innervate the bronchial tubes.

The lungs fill the thoracic cavity. The back, sternum, and ribs encase the whole lung. During inspiration the top of the lung extends to the first rib and the bottom of the lung to the tenth rib.

The right lung has three lobes while the left has two. The right lung has an upper and lower lobe separated by the major fissure and a middle lobe separated from the upper lobe by the horizontal fissure. The left lung has an upper lobe separated from the lower lobe by the major fissure.

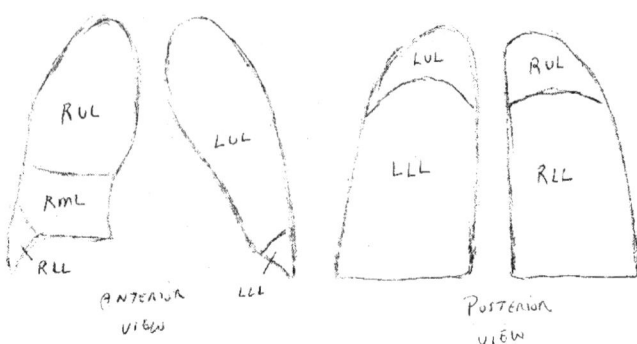

RUL is the right upper lobe, RML the middle lobe, RLL is the RLL. LUL is the left upper lobe and LLL is the left lower lobe

The most important thing to remember is that when we listen to the back of the chest we are listening mainly to the lower lobe. When we listen to the front of the chest we are listening to mainly the upper lobe on the left side, and the upper lobe and middle lobe on the right side.

The lobes are further divided into segments. There are ten segments in the right lung and eight in the left lung.

The segments of the right lung include the apical, posterior, and anterior segments of the right upper lobe, the lateral and medial segments of the middle lobe, and the superior, medial basal, anterior basal, lateral basal and posterior basal of the right lower lobe.

The segments in the left lung include the apical/posterior, anterior, superior lingula, and inferior lingula of the left upper lobe as well as the superior, anterior medial basal, lateral basal and posterior basal of the left lower lobe.

The superior segments of the lower lobes are the largest segments and are located at the apex of the lower lobes. They are the most common site of pneumonia.

IMPORTANT CONCEPTS TO REMEMBER FROM THIS LECTURE

1. Shingles is caused by the virus that causes

    Chicken pox

2. The Xiphoid process is

    A cartilage located at the very bottom of the sternum that projects into the upper abdomen

3. The diaphragm is innervated by the

    Phrenic nerve which is innervated by the 3rd, 4th and 5th cervical nerve roots

4. The accessory muscles of inspiration include the:

    External Intercostal muscles, Scalene muscles, Sternocleidomastoid muscles, Pectoralis major muscles, and the Trapezius muscles

5. The Visceral Pleura has pain receptors?

    False

6. When we listen to the back of the chest most of what we hear is from the:

    Lower lobes

Lecture Nine

The Lower Airways

The lung consists of two functional units, the airways which are the tubes that bring oxygen and carbon dioxide into and out of the lungs and the parenchyma including the respiratory bronchioles, the alveolar ducts and the alveoli where gas exchange between the outside world and the blood actually takes place. The airways consist of a series of ever smaller, ever simpler but ever more numerous tubes. The airways start at the bottom of the larynx with the trachea and end at the alveoli. There are about 450,000,000 tiny air sacs or alveoli, each sac engulfed by myriads of capillaries. Their total surface area is 75 square meters or about 700 square feet.

The Airways

Many texts divide the airways into groups based on their characteristics such as whether or not they contain cartilage, whether they have pseudociliated columnar epithelium or cuboidal epithelium, and whether or not they have smooth muscle. I think it is more physiologic to classify airways by studying how they move oxygen and carbon dioxide. The largest airways, like the trachea, bronchi, and non-respiratory bronchioles, move air by mass transport which is similar to how the air comes out between your lips when you try to blow out a candle. The smallest airways, on the other hand, are so numerous that the sum of their cross-sectional area is huge. It would be like standing at the far end of the table when your little one, at the other end, bends over the cake and blows out the candles. You won't feel any blast of air at your end at all.

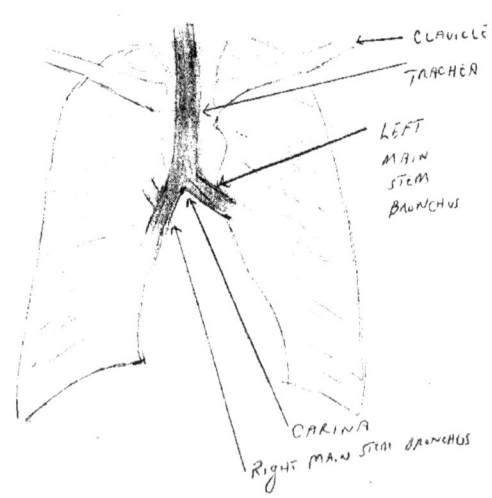

The trachea divides into the right and left main stem bronchi. The division is called the carina.

The trachea is the largest airway. It begins just below the cricoid cartilage of the larynx. It is a large U-shaped (or C-shaped) tube, with the round part of the U pointed anteriorly. It is about 2.5 cm in its largest diameter and about 12 cm in length. It ends by bifurcating into the right and left main stem bronchi just behind the Angle of Louis of the sternum. You can palpate your trachea if you place your finger in the sternal notch. The trachea should always be in the midline. The bifurcation of the trachea is called the *carina* because when you look at it through a bronchoscope it is shaped like the bow of a ship.

The right main stem bronchus arises at an angle of about 30 degrees from the midline while the left main stem bronchus arises at a much more horizontal angle of about 60 degrees. Thus if you accidently inhale a peanut, it is a lot easier for the peanut to roll down into your right main stem bronchus than into your left main stem bronchus. Like the trachea the main stem bronchi are U-shaped.

Arising from the main stem bronchi are the lobar bronchi which branch into the segmental bronchi. These branch into the subsegmental bronchi which branch into the bronchioles, which branch into the terminal bronchioles. Up to this point, the movement of air is by *mass movement*. In other words, inspiration creates a negative pressure in the chest which forces air to move from the trachea all the way down to the terminal bronchioles. But by the level of the terminal bronchioles, even though the size of each airway is very small, there are so many of these tiny airways that their total cross-sectional area has become huge and air flow becomes nearly negligible.

The cross-sectional area of the trachea is about 2.5 cm^2. The cross-sectional area of the bronchi remains about the same unti the 5th division, or about the level of the subsegmental airways, then the cross-sectional area increases exponentially so that by the 10th generation of bronchioles it is about 20 cm^2. By the 15th generation it is about 150 cm^2 and by the 20th generation it is over 1400 cm^2. That is about one square meter!

The last three generations of airways are called the *respiratory zone* because alveoli can arise from their walls and gas exchange can occur. These last generations are sometimes called the "primary lobule". The respiratory bronchioles divide into the alveolar ducts, which finally come to an end in the alveolar sacs. The transport of gases such as oxygen and carbon dioxide in this part of the lung is by *diffusion*.

The trachea is U or C shaped because it has cartilage on three sides which support its structure. The cartilage is located on the anterior and lateral surfaces of the tubing. The back wall of the trachea is membranous and is adjacent to the flattened esophagus located just behind it. The main stem bronchi have a similar structure.

The bronchioles are the small airways. They are only about one-half of a millimeter in diameter. They are surrounded by smooth muscle and are compressible. That means when you breathe in they dilate and when you exhale they collapse. The small airways are lined by cuboidal cells. The cilia have disappeared, but they may still have glands, although these too are becoming less and less frequent.

The structure becomes more complex in the respiratory bronchioles. Alveolar sacs appear in the wall of the bronchioles. Canals of Lambert, which connect respiratory bronchioles with alveoli begin to be seen as well. These canals, like the pores of Kohn which connect alveolus to alveolus, probably function as collateral ventilation for the alveoli to aid gas exchange and prevent atelectasis.

In addition Club Cells or Bronchiolar Exocrine Cells or, as they once were known as, Clara Cells[1], appear in the wall of the bronchioles as the goblet cells disappear. These are dome-shaped, cuboidal cells without microvilli. These cells secrete glycoproteinaceous chemicals which function to protect the airways. They also secrete enzymes which help protect the airways against foreign invaders.

Mucociliary Ladder[2]

The cilia lining the large airways are bathed in a two-layered mucous fluid. In the past the mucous was divided into a "sol" solution bathing the cilia, and a "gel" layer located above the cilia. It is now certain that there are two "gel" layers instead. There is a mucous layer and a periciliary layer instead. The periciliary layer has a higher osmotic pressure helping to maintain better hydration in healthy people and therefor better transport of the thicker mucous layer above.

Mucous travels at about 50 micrometers per second from the distal airways to the trachea. Mucous that reaches the trachea can be coughed up. Mucous in the small airways can't. In the small airways the mucous accumulates providing a site for infection.

Mucous consists of 98% water, 0.9% salt, .8% globular protein, and 0.3% high molecular weight mucin polymers. It is the latter which is most important because these proteins form a mesh-like gel. The more concentrated the mucous the thicker the gel and the slower the mucociliary ladder. Thus dehydration of the mucous layer is an important component of several diseases and treatment must be directed at rehydration of this layer. This is the reason that hypertonic saline inhalations are so important in Cystic Fibrosis.

When the mucociliary layer fails diseases such as bronchiectasis and exacerbations of chronic obstructive disease may be the result.

The blood supply for the airways is not from the pulmonary arteries but from the bronchial arteries which arise directly from the aorta. Only the tiny respiratory airways, alveolar ducts, and alveoli receive their blood supply from a combination of the bronchial arteries and pulmonary arteries. The bronchial arteries also supply the esophagus and pleura. The bronchial veins drain the bronchi, esophagus, and pleura.

The bronchi are innervated by the sympathetic and parasympathetic nervous systems. There are no pain fibers at all!

Histologically, the trachea and main stem bronchi are lined by pseudostratified ciliated columnar epithelium. The lining is called "pseudostratified" because while it looks like there are several layers of columnar epithelium there is actually just one layer. Each columnar cell arises from the basement membrane. Interspersed amongst the columnar cells are goblet cells, which secrete mucous. The Kulchinsky Cell, a granular cell, is found along the basement membrane as well. These cells are neuroendocrine cells and are quite hormonally active. They are derived from the

---

[1] Clara Cells were first discovered by Max Clara in 1937. He was a Nazi who conducted experiments on prisoners executed by the Nazi regime. In May of 2012, the editorial boards of many international pulmonary journals renamed the Clara Cells so as not to honor the man. The change in name took effect January 1, 2013.
[2] Richard Boucher, Muco-Obstructive Lung Diseases, NEJM 2019, 380: 1941-53

primitive spinal cord, called the *notochord*. They give rise to a very malignant tumor, called the *small cell cancer* or "oat cell" cancer in smokers.

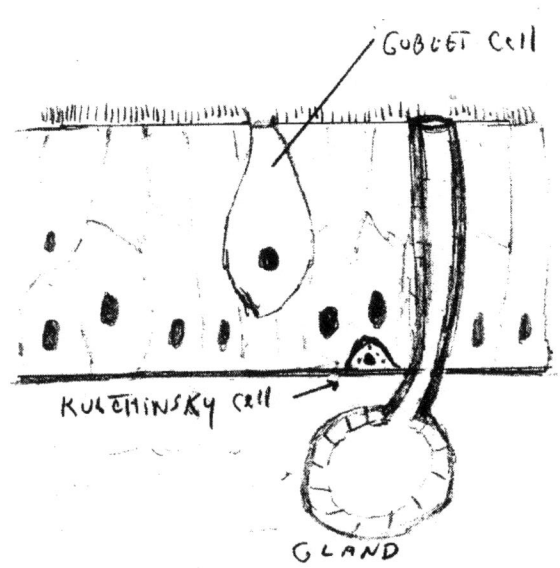

Pseudostratified Ciliated Columnar epithelium

As division after division occurs and the airways get smaller and smaller, they become simpler histologically. The cartilage is the first to disappear, then the glands. Finally, the epithelium consists of single layer of cuboidal cells lying over a basement membrane. Since there are no glands or goblet cells, the Club Cells must provide the lubrication and protection for the epithelium of these tiny airways.

The Lung Parenchyma

The movement of oxygen and other gases in the parenchyma of the lung is by diffusion *at least during quiet breathing*. Diffusion is the movement of a molecule from an area of high concentration to an area of low concentration because of the random movement of the gas. We will spend one entire lecture discussing diffusion shortly. There is evidence, however, in mice that with greater changes in lung volumes, the alveoli expand with inhalation, in part due to recruitment of additional alveoli because of the cross-ventilation through Pores of Kohn, and collapse with exhalation. Thus with large breaths there still may be some mass movement of gases in the parenchyma of the lung.

The word "alveolus" comes from the Latin and means "little cavity". The alveolus is a sac-like, air-filled structure which is encased in a web of tiny capillaries. It is about .2 micrometers in diameter and about 4 cubic micrometers in volume. Interestingly, total lung volume correlates with number of alveoli.

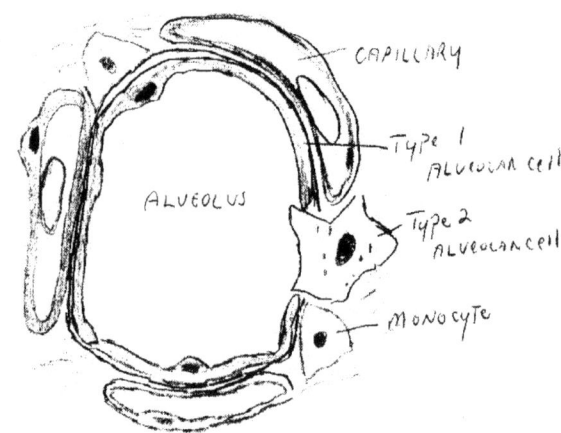

A schematic of the alveolus showing the relationship of the alveolus to the capillaries as well as the three types of cells found in the alveolus: the alveolar type 1, alveolar type 2, and the monocyte (macrophage)

The alveolus has a single layer of epithelium, called the Alveolar Type 1 cell, which is separated from a dense basement membrane by a thin band of fibrous tissue. On the other side of the basement membrane is another band of connective tissue then the capillary endothelium, which, like the alveolus, is composed of only a single layer of endothelial cells. Type 2 Alveolar Cells, which produce surfactant, are located at the corners of the alveolus. The alveoli also contain numerous macrophages.

The type 1 alveolar cells are thin, flat cells that form 95% of the surface of the alveoli. These cells are derived from the type 2 alveolar cells which can convert to type 1 alveolar cells when needed. The type 1 cells are the primary site for gas exchange.

The type 2 alveolar cells are cuboidal in shape and have microvilli. They manufacture and secrete surfactant, which is the chemical that lowers surface tension so that the alveoli don't collapse every time we exhale.

The alveolar macrophages are derived from the blood monocyte and are scavengers which destroy foreign invaders, such as bacteria, that manage to make it all the way to the alveolus.

The distance a molecule of oxygen has to travel from inside the alveolus to inside the capillary is less than 2.5 micra[3], one third the diameter of a red blood cell.

The lymphatics of the lung

The lymphatic channels are important. As discussed in the section on circulation, when the interstitial tissue of the lung becomes saturated with fluid, it is the lymphatics which channel the fluid into larger and larger tubes which ultimately form the *thoracic duct* which returns the fluid to the

---

[2] One study comparing low-landers and high-landers found that the alveolar-capillary membrane was only 0.65 micra.

blood where the *thoracic duct* drains into the left brachiocephalic vein. Anatomically, this is where the left subclavian vein and left internal carotid vein merge. Because of that, a lung cancer, even a lung cancer in the right lower lobe, may present with a large swollen gland in the left supraclavicular space. The swollen cancerous lymph node is called Virchow's node. The thoracic duct transports up to four liters of lymph fluid a day!

Most of the larger lymph channels are found underlying the visceral pleura as well as in the interstitial tissue surrounding the bronchi, pulmonary arteries, and pulmonary veins. Some of the larger channels actually have bands of smooth muscle which help squeeze the fluid from inside the lung towards the large lymph channels in the hilum of the lung.

There are lymph nodes widely dispersed along the lymph channels which act as filters. They help prevent bacteria and other foreign invaders getting from the lung into the blood stream via the lymph channels.

The Neural Control of the Airways

The autonomic nervous system acts on the bronchial tubes to maintain the tone of the airways. We will discuss the neural control in the lecture about "Control of Ventilation" in Lecture 15.

IMPORTANT CONCEPTS TO REMEMBER FROM THIS LECTURE

1. The trachea is lined by what type of epithelium?
   Pseudostratified ciliated columnar epithelium

2. What are Kulchinsky cells?
   Neuroendocrine cells derived from the primitive spinal cord called the notochord.

3. What are Club Cells?
   Club cells are found in the terminal and respiratory bronchioles. They secrete proteins and enzymes which protect the epithelium of the airways as well as attack foreign invaders.

4. Where do Alveolar Type 1 cells arise from?
   Alveolar Type 2 cells both secrete surfactant and give rise when needed to Alveolar Type 1 Cells.

5. Where do the Alveolar Macrophages come from?
   The Monocytes found in the blood

Lecture Ten

Static Properties of the Lung

In the last lecture we split the lungs into two compartments, the airways made up of the trachea, bronchi and bronchioles and the lung parenchyma made up of the alveoli, capillaries, and the supporting interstitial tissues. We need to exam each of the compartments separately because they are so different. The airways transport oxygen and carbon dioxide by mass movement and their parameters are Pressure and Flow. In contrast movement of oxygen and carbon dioxide in the lung parenchyma is due to the random movement of molecules or Brownian movement. In addition, the parenchyma must expand and contract with changes in the pleural pressure. Thusly, its parameters are Pressure and Volume. Even the manifestations of disease differ between the two compartments. Disease of the airways generally causes obstructive lung disease and disease of the lung parenchyma generally causes restrictive lung disease.

When we inhale, our diaphragm and external intercostal muscles contract enlarging our thorax, creating a negative pressure in our pleural space. Since the pressure in our pleural space is less than atmospheric pressure, so long as our mouth and glottis are open, air will flow from our mouth into our alveoli. This sounds so very simple.

But at least two things are involved in this process. The lungs must expand overcoming the elastic properties of the lung and air must flow overcoming the resistance of the tubing. Thus the force of inspiration must do two things:

Force (pressure) is proportional to the change in volume and change in flow

We will look at each part of the equation: the change in volume and the change in flow. The change in volume is described by the static properties of the lung and the change in flow is described by the dynamic properties of the lung. This lecture will focus on the static properties.

Ventilation is the process in which carbon dioxide is moved from the alveolus to the external environment and oxygen is moved from the external environment into the alveolus. It has two components. The mass flow of gases, which occurs in the large airways, such as the trachea and bronchial tubes and Brownian movement, which is the random movement of molecules or gases along a pressure gradient. This occurs in the smallest airways.

Both mass flow and Brownian movement are driven by the difference in pressures between two areas, whether it is the difference in pressure between the mouth and the small airways in mass flow seen in the bronchial tubes or the difference in the partial pressure of oxygen and carbon dioxide between the alveoli and the capillaries.

What is pressure? Pressure is a continuous physical force exerted on or against an object by something in contact with it. Force (pressure) equals Mass X Acceleration. The greater the force the faster we can make a given mass move.

When we speak of *atmospheric pressure* we are talking about how much force the atmosphere is pushing down on our heads. At sea level it is about 760 mm of mercury or 1033 cm H_2O. On the top of Mount Everest it is much less. In fact it is 1/3rd of the atmospheric pressure at sea level or about 253 mm Hg. At the bottom of Death Valley, it is about 5% higher than sea level because there is more atmosphere above us.

We will always compare the pressures we measure to atmospheric pressure.

For inspiration to occur, the pressure in the alveoli must always be less than the pressure at the mouth just as when water flows from a faucet, the pressure at the mouth of the faucet must be less than the pressure in the water tank from whence the water comes. This is the major reason you don't want to build your house on a very high hill.

When you breathe in, the diaphragm contracts, the pressure in the pleural space falls, and, if the mouth and glottis are open, air rushes in. THIS IS NOT BOYLE's LAW! Boyle's law applies only to a **closed system**.

Boyle's law relates the pressure and volume in a **closed system**. Imagine we have a cylinder one liter in size that starts with a pressure of 760 mm Hg. If we compress the cylinder to half its size the pressure must double.

$$Pressure_1 \times Volume_1 = Pressure_2 \times Volume_2$$

$$760 \text{ mm Hg times } 1000 \text{ cc} = x \text{ times } 500 \text{ cc}$$

$$x = (760 \times 1000)/500 = 1520 \text{ mm Hg}$$

When we breathe in, the lungs are an **open system** and will increase in size. There is a linear relationship between pressure and lung volume.

Change in Volume = Change in Pressure X Compliance

What is compliance? Compliance is a measure of how stretchable the lungs are. The more the lungs can stretch, the greater their compliance. When we think about the compliance we often compare compliance to stretching a rubber band. The greater force we use stretching the rubber band the longer it gets. But if the rubber band is more compliant or stretchable, less force will be needed to stretch it. Think of compliance as *stretchability*. Elasticity is the inverse of compliance. It is 1/compliance.

It is better to compare the lungs to a big balloon. When we begin to blow up a balloon, we need to use a lot of force at first. Then, almost magically, only a little force is required to blow the balloon to a large volume. Finally, when the balloon is almost fully inflated it gets harder and harder to blow up the balloon. Thus a typical balloon behaves as if it has three different compliances.

The more tissue in the lung whether it be cells, water, or scarring, the stiffer they become and the less stretchable. An example would be a patient with pulmonary fibrosis, where the lung is replaced by scar tissue. On the other hand, the less elastic tissue in the lung, the more stretchable the lungs. An example would ba a patient with emphysema.

We can solve our equation relating pressure and volume for compliance and we find:

Compliance = Change in Volume/Change in Pressure

Or

C = dV/dP

But the lung exists inside a large container which we call the chest wall or thorax and both the chest wall and the lungs have an independent compliance. If we open the thorax we find that the lung collapses, just like a balloon, but the chest wall expands.

Moreover, if we include both the lung and chest wall together to measure compliance we are measuring the compliance of the total respiratory system.

In order to calculate lung, chest wall and total respiratory system compliance we must understand the different pressure gradients in the lung and how those different pressures relate to each other.

There are four pressures we must understand:

1. Oral pressure is the pressure at the open mouth. Normally this is the atmospheric pressure, but if the patient is intubated or his mouth attached to a valve which can open and close, the pressure is NOT atmospheric and it must be measured.

2. Alveolar Pressure is the pressure in the alveoli.

3. Pleural Pressure is the pressure inside the pleural space. This pressure is measured by placing a balloon pressure gauge in the esophagus which actually lies in the pleural space

4. The atmospheric pressure or the pressure outside the chest wall.

From these pressures, we can measure certain **"pressure gradients"**. The pressure difference or gradient between the mouth and the alveolus is the *transairway pressure*. The pressure gradient between the alveolar pressure and the pleural pressure is the *transpulmonary pressure*. The pressure gradient between the pleural pressure and the atmospheric pressure outside the chest wall is the *transthoracic pressure* and the pressure gradient between the atmospheric pressure and the oral pressure is the *transrespiratory pressure*.

When we compare the change in lung volume to the different pressure gradients we are actually measuring different things. If we compare the change in volume to the change in the transpulmonary pressure we are measuring the lung compliance but if we compare the change in volume to the change in transrespiratory pressure we are measuring the total respiratory system compliance.

We often report *lung compliance* on the records of intubated patients in the ICU but we never actually measure the pleural pressure. Rather we compare oral pressure to atmospheric pressure and are, in fact, measuring the total system or *respiratory system compliance*.

There is one more important concept that respiratory therapists need to understand and that is the difference between *static* compliance and *dynamic* compliance.

Static compliance is generally measured in the laboratory setting. The patient is asked to hold his breath with his mouth and glottis open while his oral pressure and pleural pressure are measured at different lung volumes. If there is **no airflow** then **the pressure at the mouth is the same as the pressure in the alveolus**.

Dynamic compliance is measured at the bedside in a patient on the ventilator. While we do pause the patient's respiration, there is still some air movement in the lungs, often just between lobes. We would have to hold the patient's breathe for many seconds to make it a truly static measurement. Dynamic compliance thus includes a component of air flow and hence resistance of the tubing and airways.

In order to measure lung compliance, we must relate the lung volume to the transpulmonary pressure (the pressure difference between the pleural space and the alveolus). We first have the patient swallow a balloon attached to a pressure sensor. The balloon lies in the esophagus which is, as you know, in the pleural space first directly behind the trachea and then in the lower part of the thorax behind the heart. We position the esophageal balloon to makes sure it is in the lower thorax. We then have the patient breathe in and hold his breath with his glottis open. When there is no airflow, the pressure at the mouth must equal the pressure inside the alveoli. We then compare the mouth or oral pressure to the pleural pressure to get the transpulmonary pressure, which we relate to the lung volume. The patient breathes out some air and we again make the measurement. We repeat the procedure till the patient exhales all the air out that he can.

While we are measuring the patient's lung compliance we can also measure his transthoracic compliance by comparing the pleural pressure to atmospheric pressure at the same time.

> **Performing the compliance measurement:**
>
> The patient first swallows an esophageal balloon in order to measure the pleural pressure (P_{pl}). Then he is connected to a spirometer in order to measure lung volumes. There is a valve to stop his respiration and a gauge to measure his oral pressure (P_o). The patient takes a deep breath and then the valve is closed and the measurements taken of his lung volume, oral and pleural pressure. This is repeated as the patient exhales stepwise to his residual volume.

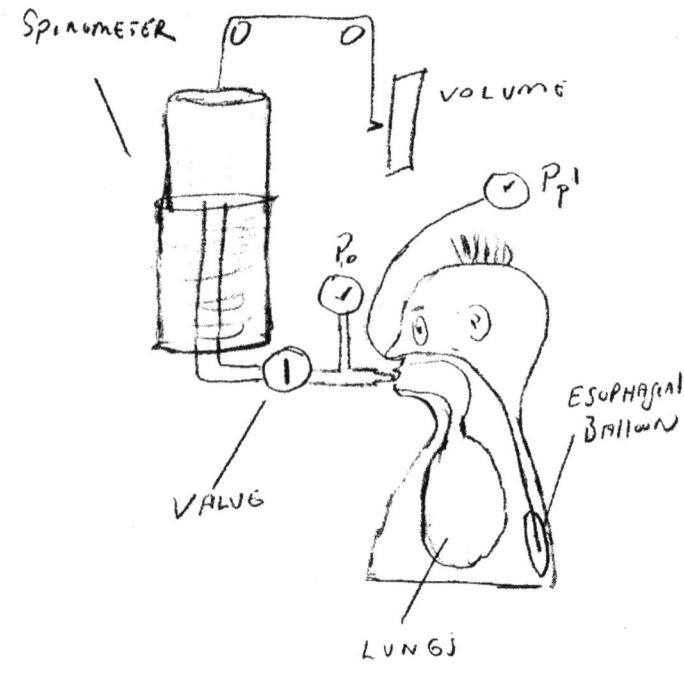

Performing a Static Compliance Measurement in the Laboratory

One of the most important pulmonary measurements is the Functional Residual Capacity (FRC). It is defined as *the amount of air in the chest at the end of a passive exhalation.* But a quick glance at the compliance curve for the lungs and chest wall shows that the FRC can be better defined as *the lung volume at which the tendency of the lungs to collapse is exactly balanced by the tendency of the chest wall to expand.* That means that at FRC the diaphragm and chest wall muscles are all at rest. The body expends no energy in maintaining the FRC.

The normal lung compliance is about 0.2 liters per cm and the normal chest wall compliance is also 0.2 liters per cm. In other words if you go from a pleural pressure of -5 to -10 you will increase your lung volume (and chest volume) by 1 liter. Because the curve for the respiratory system is much flatter, its compliance is half that of the lung compliance or about 0.1 liter per cm.

Another quick look at the curves show that for the lung volumes within a liter or so of the FRC, the compliance curves are fairly perpendicular which means that *for a small change in pressure there is a relatively large change in volume.* Thus, in the range of lung volumes near the FRC, the compliance of the lung is high. This means that the work of breathing is minimal. The oxygen cost of quiet breathing is extremely low. In fact, despite the size of the lungs and thorax, breathing only requires about 2% of the cardiac output. Compare that to the brain which requires 20% of the cardiac output.

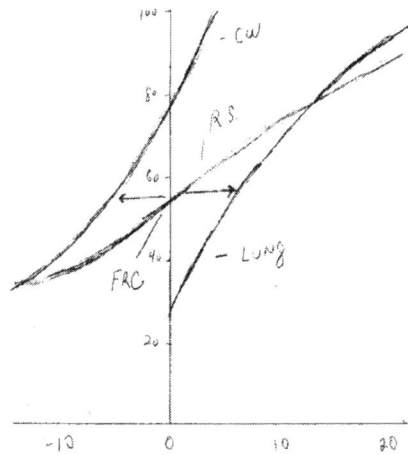

Comparing the chest wall compliance curve (CW) to the lung compliance curve shows that at about 55% of the vital capacity or 40% of the total lung capacity, the tendency of the CW to expand is exactly balance by the tendency of the lungs to collapse. This is the FRC or Functional Residual Capacity.

What diseases affect the lung's compliance? The compliance can either be reduced, which means the lungs are stiffer or it can be increased which means the lungs expand easier.

The compliance is increased (the lungs are more distensible) in emphysema due to the loss of the elastic supporting tissue of the lungs.

The compliance is decreased (the lungs are stiff) when the lungs are filled with fluid or when they are fibrosed (scarred). In addition, in newborns and in some patients with the Acute Respiratory Distress Syndrome (ARDS), there is not enough surfactant and the lungs are stiff. Surfactant is a protein containing a phospholipid group which is part water soluble because of its protein and its many charges (amino groups and carboxyl groups) and part water insoluble because of the lipid component. Surfactant lowers the surface tension making it easier to expand the lungs.

What is surface tension? Surface tension is a force on the surface of a body, whether liquid or solid, created by molecules located below the surface, which seeks to maintain the smallest surface area. It is the force which allows certain insects called "water striders" to literally walk on water. It is the force which makes liquids, such as water, form semi-spherical shapes on polished wood when one of our children spills his glassful at supper.

Water is certainly one of the best examples of surface tension because water is a "charged" molecule. It has a positive side (the two hydrogen ions) and a negative side (the oxygen). Thus, when spilled on the table, these molecules attract each other, bunch up, and form well-defined globs. The water molecules exert their force in all directions but the surface molecules have no water above them. They are drawn inward towards the center of the glob.

The effect of surface tension on the alveoli is to shrink them to the smallest size possible. Surfactant, produced by the alveolar type 2 cells, prevents the shrinkage by interacting directly with the liquid on the surface of the alveolar cells. Thus, we don't collapse our lungs every time we exhale.

As we inhale, the alveoli get larger and surfactant is diluted. But because of Laplace's Law the lungs don't suddenly collapse.

Laplace's Law states that the pressure needed to distend a balloon is equal to a constant multiplied by the surface tension of the balloon divided by its radius.

Pressure = K times Surface tension/radius

Thus if the surface tension is high, a lot of force will be needed to blow up the balloon. On the other hand if the surface tension is low, less force will be needed. Changes in the radius of the balloon are more important however. As the balloon gets bigger, its radius gets bigger, and the pressure needed to blow up the balloon gets less and less. Remember when you blew up your child's balloon at his or her last birthday. It was very hard to get the balloon inflated at first, but once you got it going, it got easier and easier. You can thank Laplace for this.

Thus at FRC, the alveoli in the lower lobe are small. Without surfactant they would be hard to fill with air. Surfactant is in high concentration at FRC. As the alveoli expand, the surfactant concentration decreases but Laplace's law takes over. It gets easier and easier to expand the alveoli because the radii of the alveoli are getting larger and larger.

How effective is surfactant? It reduces the surface tension by 80% from 50 dynes/cm to 10 dynes/cm.

Surfactant levels are markedly reduced in infants born prematurely who often develop a condition called "Hyaline Membrane Disease" or the "Respiratory Distress Syndrome". The treatment is to replace the surfactant. Cortisone is also given to the mother before delivery to stimulate the Type 2 Alveolar cells to produce surfactant.

The Acute Respiratory Distress Syndrome which is seen in patients with sepsis or shock from other causes has a similar pathology to the "Respiratory Distress Syndrome" seen in children. Surfactant has been tried but has not been shown to be effective.

Surfactant is decreased by acidosis, hypoxia, hyperoxia, atelectasis, and pulmonary vascular congestion.

Lecture Notes: Anatomy and Physiology for the Respiratory Therapist

IMPORTANT CONCEPTS TO REMEMBER FROM THIS LECTURE

1. Boyle's Law states that:

    In a closed system, $P_1V_1 = P_2V_2$

2. Transpulmonary pressure is the:

    Pressure across the lungs (from inside the alveolus to the pleural space)

3. The Lung Compliance is the:

    Change in lung volume related to the change in transpulmonary pressure.

4. When a patient is on a ventilator we measure his or her:

    Total respiratory compliance **NOT** the lung compliance.

5. Laplace's Law States:

    The force needed to expand a balloon equals a constant times the surface tension divided by the radius of the balloon.

Lecture Eleven

Dynamic Properties of the Lung

The lung is not just an elastic balloon which expands and contracts. Air, carrying oxygen into and carbon dioxide out of the body, flows in and out of our lungs for as long as we walk on the earth. But what factors affect the air flow?

We might compare our airways to the pipes in a new home. What factors will affect the flow of water in our faucets? If we only get a drip, drip, drip when we shower what can we do to make the flow better?

The most obvious factor is the size of the pipes. Are they half-inch in diameter or three-quarter-inches in diameter? Even the water company knows you get a lot more water with a bigger pipe. They charge a lot more for a connection to a larger pipe. What about how long the pipe is? If you are the last house getting water from the water system it may be a reason to move. But I think we all realize that this, intuitively, is not as important as the diameter of the pipe.

If you have a house on a very tall hill, say a hill 50 feet tall and the water tower that supplies your house is 60 feet up, you are not going to get as much water as someone living fifty feet below you in the valley. The pressure gradient at your house is 60 – 50 or 10, while at the house at the bottom of the hill it is 60 – 0 or 60. Your friend, whom you love to look down on, is going to enjoy his shower a lot more than you will.

Other factors might include obstructions in the piping. But these are more akin to diseases of the pipe and not to the underlying physiology.

From our considerations, simple though they may seem to be, we can conclude that:

Flow is proportional to the size of the tube and the driving force and inversely related to the length of the tubing.

The driving force for air flow is the pressure gradient. Air flows from an area of high pressure to an area of low pressure. Flow **only** occurs when there is a pressure gradient. There is no gas flow when the pressure between two points is equal, i.e., when the faucet is closed the pressure is the same throughout the pipe and water will not flow. *The movement of a liquid or gas is always from an area of high pressure to an area of low pressure.*

Pressure equals the flow multiplied by the resistance:

Pressure = Flow X resistance

Solving for flow we get:

Flow = Pressure / Resistance

Flow is the movement of a liquid or gas. It is like the velocity of a car or wind speed.

Poiseuille's law (pronounced PWAAZ EE) expands the Resistance in our equation. It states that the radius of the tube affects the flow even more than the pressure. If the pressure doubles, the flow doubles.

Resistance = K times 8 times length of the tube X viscosity/Radius to the 4th power.

The radius is in the denominator. **Therefore, the larger the tube the smaller the resistance**. On the other hand, the smaller the tube, the greater the resistance and the slower the flow at any given pressure. If the radius of the tube doubles, the flow increases 16 fold (2 X 2 X 2 X 2).

Putting *Poiseuille's law* into our equation for flow we get:

Flow = Pressure X Radius to the fourth power X Pi/ 8 X length of the tube X viscosity

But Poiseuille's law only applies to laminar flow. Laminar flow is smooth, linear flow. Gas travels in parallel straight lines, the fastest molecules in the center of the stream, the slowest near the wall of the tube.

If the flow is turbulent, meaning there are a lot of twists and turns and little cyclones, called *Eddy Currents*, Poiseuille's law no longer applies and the resistance to flow is much greater.

With quiet breathing the flow though our airways is probably all laminar flow. But during a cough or rapid, deep breathing the flow in the larger airways becomes turbulent and some extra force must be wasted on overcoming the increased resistance.

Time Constants:

The last concept we need to discuss at this point is the idea of "time constants." The time constant is the time required to deflate a part of the lung to 63% of its maximum volume. It is defined in the following equation:

Time constant = resistance X compliance

If the resistance doubles, the time constant will double. Thus the patient will require more time to inflate the lungs. The faster the patient breathes the less air he will get. For that patient it is better to breathe slow and deep.

On the other hand, if a patient has stiff lungs, the compliance will decrease and the time constant will be less. It will take less time to inflate and deflate the lungs. But because the lungs are stiffer, the maximum inhaled volume will be decreased out of proportion to the change in the time constant. The patient with stiff lungs will need to hyperventilate with low lung volumes.

Obstructive Airways Disease is caused by two different mechanisms. The first is physical obstruction of the airway itself because the airways are narrowed or a filled with debris such as mucous. The second is more interesting. The airways are collapsible tubes. When we exhale forcibly, the pleural pressure increases and, if the elastic supporting structure of the airways is weakened or if the cartilaginous walls of the airway are weak, the airways will collapse. Inspiratory flows will be near normal or normal but expiratory flows will be reduced. The first condition is, of course, emphysema. The second is a condition called chondromalacia which is a hereditary disease in which the cartilage is more like paper than plastic.

Common Ventilatory Patterns.

Breathing has two components: frequency and depth of respiration. We think of the normal breathing rate as about 16 and the normal tidal volume as about 500 cc. The value for the normal breathing rate was found observing people sitting comfortably at a church service. There is normally a pause at the end of exhalation so that the ratio between time of inspiration and the time of expiration is about 1:2. In other words expiration is twice as long as inspiration.

The average rate of breathing varies with age. The newborn breathes about 30-60 times a minute, the toddler about 25-40, the child about 20-30 and the adult about 12-20.

We have already mentioned that because of changes in the time constant the patient with mild asthma or COPD will have an increased tidal volume and decreased frequency while the patient with pulmonary fibrosis will have a decreased tidal volume and increased frequency.

When we discuss breathing patterns and ventilation we must be sure we are talking about the same thing. Not all the air we breathe gets down to the alveoli. Some just ventilates the major airways like the trachea and large bronchi. This is called dead space ventilation. It has nothing to do with gas exchange. In some diseases the dead space ventilation increases dramatically because of changes in the relationship between blood flow and ventilation as we will see in the next lecture. These patients can have a large total ventilation but a very small alveolar ventilation. It is imperative that you understand when you are describing ventilation whether you are talking about total ventilation which is the movement of air at the mouth, or alveolar ventilation which is the amount of air that is actually involved in gas exchange. Importantly, the alveolar ventilation is inversely related to the pCO_2 in the blood. The greater the alveolar ventilation the lower the pCO_2. Decreasing alveolar ventilation increases the pCO_2. A patient with severe asthma, can come to the emergency room breathing very fast and struggling to breathe faster, but his or her pCO_2 may be very high, because the alveolar ventilation is very low because of their large dead space ventilation.

There are several different patterns of breathing that are well described:

Apnea means the absence of any breathing.

Eupnea is the normal breathing pattern.

Hyperpnoea means to take deep breaths.

Tachypnea means to breathe faster.

Hyperventilation means to breathe faster and deeper. It is often associated with stress or exercise.

Bradypnea means to breathe slower.

Hypoventilation means decreased rate and depth of breathing

Biot's Respiration is characterized by bouts of extremely deep and fast respiration alternating with apneic spells. This is often seen in patients who have meningitis or who have had a stroke.

Cheyne-Stokes respiration is characterized by a cyclic pattern of respiration. The patient has periods of apnea followed by ever increasing tidal breaths till he or she reaches a maximum. Then the tidal breath decrease in volume steadily till the apnea returns. This pattern is seen most often in patients with central nervous system disease such as a stroke associated with congestive heart failure.

Kussmaul's respiration is characterized by rapid, extremely deep breathing. The patient breathes as hard and fast as he can. This is usually seen in patients with severe acidosis such as diabetic ketoacidosis, lactic acidosis (a septic patient) or renal failure.

The concept that leads to the greatest confusion for most students is differentiating between Biot's respiration and Cheyne-Stokes respiration. In Biot's the breathing alternates between deep and rapid respirations and total apnea. In Cheyne-Stokes respiration, while there is also apnea alternating with hyperventilation, the breathing has a pattern of waxing and waning rather than the abrupt onset of apnea and hyperventilation.

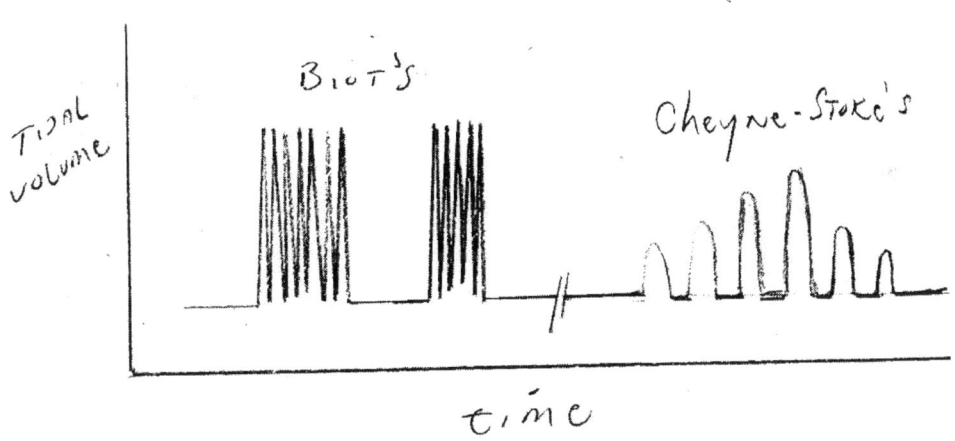

Comparing Biot's Respiration with Cheyne - Stokes respiration

IMPORTANT CONCEPTS TO REMEMBER FROM THIS LECTURE

1. Pressure equals Resistance Times?
    Flow

2. If the radius of a pipe doubles, the flow will increase by?
    The flow will increase 16 fold.

3. What is Poiseuille's law?
    It states that the pressure gradient as well as the radius and length of the tube affect the air flow. The smaller the tube, the slower the flow at any given pressure gradient. The larger the tube the greater the flow at any given pressure gradient.

4. When the compliance decreases the respiratory rate will?
    Increase

5. Biot's Respiration is characterized by?
    The respiratory pattern characterized by the abrupt onset of apnea alternating with the abrupt onset of hyperventilation

Lecture Twelve

The Relationship between Ventilation and Perfusion

The relationship between ventilation and perfusion is, to my mind, the most important concept we need to understand if we want to get a handle on why patients with pulmonary disease are hypoxemic. We will see how the effect of gravity determines the distribution of both ventilation and perfusion. It is important physiologically. It is even more important clinically.

While we often are told in our textbooks that elevated carbon dioxide levels are due to "hypoventilation", it is hard to imagine a child in the emergency room with an acute asthma attack, a carbon dioxide level of 50, and a respiratory rate of 50 actually being diagnosed with hypoxemia due to "hypoventilation" in the same sense as a patient who overdosed on heroin.

Another example, but of a totally different nature, is pulmonary fibrosis, in which parts of the lung are replaced by scar tissue. Because there is an increase in the interstitial tissue the hypoxemia is said to be due to a "diffusion block". Careful examination shows, however, that early on in the disease process, the thickened interstitial tissue is located in the areas of the alveoli that are not involved in gas transport. In both these cases the true cause of the hypoxemia is ventilation-perfusion inequality.

The effects of ventilation and perfusion inequality also explain why patients with emphysema have normal blood gases while patients with chronic bronchitis have severely abnormal blood gases.

Thus understanding the relationship between ventilation and perfusion is necessary to have any understanding of the physiology and pathology of the lung.

Intuitively, I think we all expect that ventilation and perfusion should be perfectly matched throughout the entire lung. The relationship between ventilation and perfusion in every alveolus should be 1 to 1. But this is not the case at all. There is, in fact, only one level in the whole chest of the upright person where ventilation and perfusion are exactly matched. Over the whole lung, ventilation and perfusion are perfectly aligned. There is 5,250 ml of alveolar ventilation and 5,000 ml of pulmonary blood flow per minute. But in any given segment of the lung mismatching is more likely than matching.

The mismatching occurs because of the effect of gravity. At the base of the lung the pleural pressure is about -5 mm Hg. The lung is about 20-30 cm in height. Therefore at the top of the lung the pleural pressure will be much less, about -10 to -15 mm Hg in fact.

Let us first look at ventilation. From our study of compliance we recall that lung volume, and therefore alveolar volume, is directly related to the pleural pressure. At FRC the pleural pressure is about -5 mm Hg while at Total Lung Capacity (TLC) the pleural pressure is about -30 mm Hg. Therefore at the bottom of the lung where the pleural pressure is -5 mm Hg the alveoli must be relatively small while at the top of the lung, where the pleural pressure is -15 to -20 mm Hg, the alveoli must be much larger. When we inhale most of our ventilation will go to the lower lung. The alveoli in the lower lung field have more room to expand. The alveoli in the upper lung field are already nearly filled.

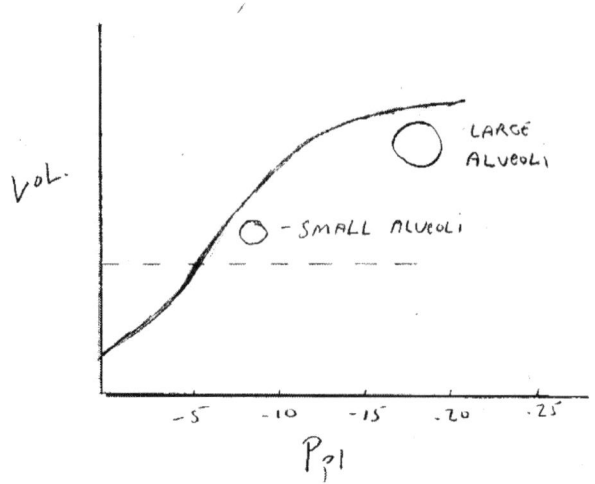

At low pleural pressures the alveoli are small and with inhalation can expand a lot. At high pleural pressures the alveoli are already distended. Thus most of inhalation goes to the lower lobes.

Gravity has a similar effect on blood flow. Blood is heavy. Thus most of the blood coming from the right ventricle goes to the lower lobes even though the pulmonary artery pressure is 10 to 12 mm Hg. Much less blood goes to the upper lobes.

John West, the great pulmonary physiologist divided the lung into three zones. At the top of the lung (Zone 1), the alveolar pressure exceeds both arterial and venous pressures. Thus, there is no blood flow. In the mid portion of the lung (zone 2), only the arterial pressure exceeds the alveolar pressure. Thus blood flow depends upon the difference between the alveolar pressure and the arterial pressure. In the lower portion of the lung (zone 3), both the arterial and venous pressures exceed the alveolar pressure and blood flow depends upon the difference between the arterial and venous pressure. Recently a zone four has been added at the very bottom of the lung. In this zone blood flow decreases because the blood vessels become compressed which increases pulmonary vascular resistance and decreases blood flow.

Because blood is much heavier than the air-filled lung, gravity has a disproportionate effect on blood flow compared to ventilation. This means that the curves for blood flow and ventilation at any given level in the chest are NOT parallel. At the top of the lung there is more ventilation than perfusion while at the bottom of the lung there is more perfusion than ventilation. The areas of the lung with a high ventilation/perfusion ratio are called areas of "dead space ventilation" while the areas with low ventilation/perfusion ratios are said to be areas of "physiologic shunting."

At the top of the lung where the ventilation/perfusion ratio is high, most of the gas in the alveoli has levels of oxygen and carbon dioxide similar to the ambient air. In other words, the alveoli have a very high oxygen level and a low carbon dioxide level.

At the bottom of the lungs, there is more blood flow. More oxygen is extracted from the alveoli and more carbon dioxide discharged into the alveoli. The oxygen level in the alveoli is only about 80 torr and the carbon dioxide is about 46.

Because the upper lung fields have relatively less blood flow they have only a minor effect on the blood gases. Thus, dead space ventilation plays a much less important role in the blood gas studies than does physiologic shunting.

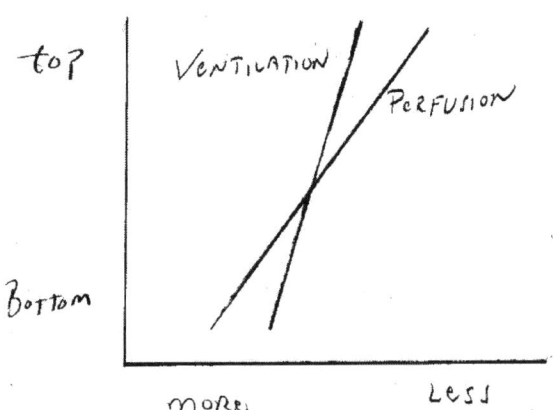

The lines for ventilation and perfusion are not parallel so that at the top of the lung there is more ventilation than perfusion (high V/Q) while at the lung basses there is more perfusion than ventilation (low V/Q). Only at one level in the lungs is the V/Q ratio equal to 1. That point is where the two lines cross.

The patient with emphysema has lost much of his or her alveoli and their accompanying capillaries. They have been destroyed. Instead of tiny alveoli there are large blebs and bulla. Thus there is more dead space ventilation which has little effect on the blood gases. The patient with emphysema is the "pink puffer". He breathes fast but his blood gases are normal. The patient with chronic bronchitis is the "blue bloater." Because his airways are filled with mucous and the bronchial walls are inflamed, he has more physiologic shunting and his oxygen level is quite low and his carbon dioxide level high.

Most pulmonary diseases, such as asthma, will cause both increased dead space ventilation and physiologic shunting. Some pulmonary diseases cause more specific changes. Pulmonary diseases which mainly increase the V/Q ratio include pulmonary emboli (early on in the course of the disease before histamines are released which cause bronchospasm), obstruction or destruction of pulmonary arteries and decreased cardiac output. The pulmonary diseases which decrease the V/Q include chronic bronchitis, bronchiectasis, some restrictive lung diseases, as well as hypoventilation.

A hallmark of hypoxemia due to V/Q inequality is that the hypoxemia responds to low flow oxygen.

Difference between Total and Alveolar Ventilation and the Bohr Equation

In our discussions about hyperventilation we stressed that total ventilation is not the same as alveolar ventilation. Total ventilation includes not only the alveolar ventilation but also the dead space ventilation. The dead space ventilation is the ventilation going to the parts of the lung that aren't perfused so that they don't participate in gas exchange.

The dead space ventilation obviously includes the anatomic dead space which consists of the large airways such as the trachea and bronchial tubes. The physiologic dead space includes the alveoli which have relatively poor perfusion with respect to their ventilation.

The total dead space is calculated by using the Bohr Equation:

$$\frac{V_d}{V_t} = \frac{P_aCO_2 - P_eCO_2}{P_aCO_2}$$

Bohr Equation

Where Vd is the dead space; Vt is the tidal volume; Little "a" stands for arterial; little "e" is expired gas.

In general the anatomic dead space is about 1 ml per pound body weight. Thus for a 120 pound woman it would be about 120 ml and for a 150 pound man it would be about 150 ml.

For example: a 150 lb. patient has a tidal volume of 600 cc, a PaCO2 of 40 and a PeCO2 of 30. What is the total dead space and the "Alveolar" dead space?

From the Bohr equation:

Vd = Vt X (PaCO2-PeCO2)/PaCO2

Vd= 600 X (40-20)/40

Vd = 600 X 20/40

Vd = 600 X .5 or 300 ml

After calculating the total dead space we have to subtract the anatomic dead space to get the alveolar dead space:

The "Alveolar" dead space is 300 ml – 150 ml or 150 ml.

Why is the alveolar dead space so important? Because the alveolar ventilation is inversely related to the pCO_2! The greater the alveolar ventilation, the lower the pCO_2. The lower the alveolar ventilation, the greater the pCO_2.

Alveolar Ventilation X pCO_2 = *constant*

That is the reason that the asthmatic patient breathing at 50 times a minute with marked increased total ventilation can have a very high pCO_2. His or her alveolar ventilation is markedly reduced. In other words the patient has a very large physiologic dead space.

The Respiratory Quotient

The respiratory quotient or RQ is the ratio between the amount of carbon dioxide produced divided by the amount of oxygen consumed. The "typical" value is about 200 ml/250 ml or 0.8 but the value is totally dependent upon the patient's diet. A high fat diet will decrease the RQ to less than .7. A high Carbohydrate diet may increase the RQ to well over 1.0.

IMPORTANT CONCEPTS TO REMEMBER FROM THIS LECTURE

1. Ventilation-perfusion inequality is the most common cause of hypoxemia and is characterized by what when compared to hypoxemia due to shunting?

   – V/Q inequality responds to low amounts of oxygen

2. Which has more effect on blood gases: physiologic shunting or dead space?

   – Physiologic shunting

3. Is both blood flow and ventilation greatest at the lung bases (Zone 3)?

   – Yes

4. Are ventilation and perfusion equal at all levels of the lungs in normal individuals?

   – No. There is only one level where they are equal

5. True or False: At FRC, the alveoli at the apex of the lung are smaller than those at the base?

   – False

Lecture Thirteen

Diffusion

If I drop a bit of red dye into a glass of water, at first it will appear as a red blob on the bottom of the glass. Several minutes later, the red blob will appear less dense and there will be a pinkish haze around it. Within an hour, the blob will be gone and the once clear water filling the glass will now be pink.

What happened? The process is called *Brownian movement*. While a glass of water looks pretty quiet and calm as if nothing at all is going on, in fact, it is teeming with activity. Electron clouds are churning and the molecules of water are jumping about expending their kinetic activity. When a blob containing millions of particles is dropped into this cauldron of activity the molecules of the water bump into the particles pushing them hither and thither. The movement is *totally random*. But because the concentration of particles in the blob of red dye is greater than the surrounding area, it is more likely that the particles will move away from the blob then move towards it. Ultimately given enough time, the particles of the blob will be distributed evenly in the glass of water. This does not mean the particles stop moving. They are just as active as before but now it is equally likely that they will move up, down, right or left.

As we noted in an earlier lecture, ventilation in the larger airways is due to the mass movement of air. But once we enter the part of the lung where gas exchange occurs, mass movement becomes negligible and the movement of gas molecules occurs because of Brownian motion, a process called *diffusion*, the movement of "individual gas molecules" from an area of high concentration to an area of low concentration.

Oxygen moves from the ambient air into the alveoli and then into the capillaries because the pO_2 in the ambient air is 150 while the pO_2 in the capillaries is only 40. Carbon Dioxide moves from the capillaries into the alveoli, and then out into the ambient air because the pCO_2 in the capillaries is 40 while the pCO_2 in air is very small indeed (0.2 mmHg). Both move along their respective concentration gradients, from areas of high concentration to areas of low concentration.

But the lungs differ from our "dye in the water" example because there is a membrane which the gases must traverse. The membrane must be "semipermeable", that is, it must allow the gases or particles to pass through but not the liquid in which the gases are found. (In reality, no membrane is perfectly semipermeable but the equations will become extremely complex if we don't make this assumption.) Oxygen must traverse the alveolar-capillary (AC) membrane to get from the alveoli to the red blood cells.

Several factors affect the rate at which oxygen and carbon dioxide can cross the AC membrane. It makes sense that greater the difference in concentration of the gas from one area to the next increases the rate of diffusion as will having a greater area available for diffusion. On the other hand, the rate of diffusion will be reduced the thicker the barrier and the larger the molecule that is being diffused.

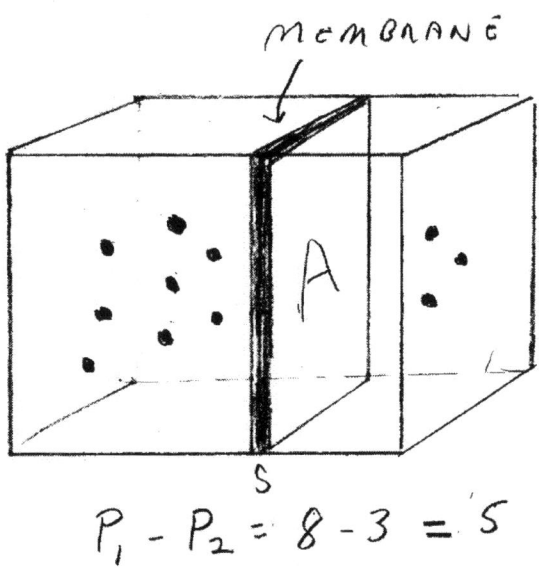

In the drawing above, A is the area of the membrane, s is the thickness of the membrane, and P1 – P2 compares the concentration of the gas on the two sides of the semipermeable membrane. Over time, the concentration of the gas will become equal on both sides of the membrane.

Thus, the rate of diffusion (dD) of a gas = a constant (K) times the partial pressure difference times the area for diffusion (A) divided by the thickness of the membrane (s).

$$dD = K \times (P1-P2) \times A/s$$

The K or constant depends directly on the type of membrane that is used. But K is also related to the size of the gas molecule and to its solubility in liquid. The larger the molecule the slower the diffusion (Graham's law). The more soluble the molecules the greater the diffusion (Henry's law). Carbon dioxide is 22 times more soluble than oxygen, but it is also heavier than oxygen. Taking both the solubility of the gases and their molecular weights into consideration, **carbon dioxide will diffuse about 20 times faster than oxygen**.

The path from the alveolus to hemoglobin is small, measuring less than 2.5 micra. Remember, the red blood cell is 7 micra in diameter so the alveolar-capillary membrane is small indeed.

From the alveolus to the hemoglobin molecule the gases must cross:

1. Liquid lining

2. Alveolar epithelial cells

3. Basement membrane of alveolar epithelial cells

4. Loose connective tissue
5. The capillary Basement membrane
6. Capillary endothelium
7. Plasma
8. Erythrocyte membrane
9. Intracellular fluid

Another factor affecting diffusion of gases in the lung is the *transit time*, which is the time a red blood cell remains in the pulmonary capillary. The transit time is a fraction of a second and during this briefest of time the red blood cell must upload oxygen and download carbon dioxide. The time between when blood enters the capillary and when it leaves is only 0.75 seconds. Exercise can decrease the transit time to as little as 0.25 seconds, 1/3rd the normal time. The good news is that oxygen uptake only requires about 0.25 seconds so that even heavy exercise won't interfere with oxygen uptake. If however, you exercise on the top of Mount Everest without oxygen, the oxygen gradient between the alveolus and the capillary will be so low that complete oxygen uptake will not occur.

What will affect the rate of diffusion? Looking at Fick's equation it is clear that anything that affects the total area of the alveolar membrane, the distance the gases have to travel from the alveolus to the capillary, and the partial pressure gradient will affect diffusion.

If the **Area** for diffusion is decreased, diffusion will be reduced. Emphysema, while considered an obstructive disease, destroys the supporting elastic tissue of the lung. Alveoli are lost as the elastic tissue is lost. Thus the area available for diffusion falls.

What about "s" or **distance**? Any disease process that causes the distance the gases have to travel from alveolus to capillary will decrease the rate of diffusion. The main culprits usually thought to cause lengthening of the distance of diffusion are the interstitial diseases such as pulmonary fibrosis, a condition in which scar tissue forms in the interstitial space surrounding the alveoli. But we know better. It is V/Q inequality instead.

Lastly, what about the **pressure gradient**. Off hand, two disorders will directly affect the pressure gradient by raising the back pressure, that is, the pressure in the capillary. The gradient is maintained, in part, because oxygen is rapidly bound to hemoglobin. But if the hemoglobin is reduced, the back pressure increases and therefore the pressure gradient is reduced as well, decreasing the rate of diffusion. Thus, anemia will cause a fall in the rate of diffusion.

A second condition that will increase the back pressure is sepsis. Remember that sepsis shuts down the mitochondria of the tissue cells. Oxygen is no longer utilized by the tissues. Thus the venous oxygen increases and the gradient between the alveolar oxygen and the capillary oxygen is reduced. This is probably not a clinical problem as the blood is completely oxygenated when it leaves the lung in the septic patient. This relationship holds so long as the patient does not have underlying lung disease such as the Acute Respiratory Distress Syndrome (ARDS).

What physiologic factors affect the rate of diffusion? The rate of diffusion decreases with age. Tall people have greater lungs volumes and hence a greater area for diffusion to occur and thus a greater rate of diffusion.

Exercise will increase the rate of diffusion. Exercise increases the pulmonary arterial blood pressure increasing the blood flow to the upper lobes. There is better matching of the air in the alveoli and the blood flow in the capillaries. In other words, the area for diffusion has increased. Lastly, when the patient is supine, diffusion is greater, probably because of better matching of alveolar ventilation and pulmonary capillary blood flow.

Dalton's Law

Dalton's law is "the law of partial pressures". **The total pressure of a gas is the sum of all the partial pressures in the gas acting independently.** Since air is made up of nitrogen, oxygen, carbon dioxide, and small amounts of other gases, the total pressure of air is the sum of the pressures of each component.

Air is made up of 78% nitrogen, 21% oxygen, 1% argon, and .03% carbon dioxide. This is true whether we are in Death Valley, CA or the very top of Mount Everest. The fiO_2 (the fraction of oxygen) is 21% at whatever altitude you are happen to be at. It is always 21%.

If we know the total pressure of air, we can calculate the pressure of each gas. If we are at sea level, the atmospheric pressure is 760 mm Hg (also called "torr"). Thus for nitrogen, 0.78 X 760 is 593 torr; for oxygen 0.21 x 760 is 160; for argon, 0.1 X 760 is 7 torr; for carbon dioxide 0.03 X 760 is 0.2 torr. But if we travel to the top of Mount Everest, the partial pressure will be only 250 mm Hg or $1/3^{rd}$ of the atmospheric pressure at sea level. Thus the pressure of its components will also be $1/3^{rd}$ of their values at sea level. For example, the partial pressure of oxygen will be 250 X .21 or 52 torr!

Remember that the partial pressure of a gas is affected by altitude but not the fraction or percentage of the gas, which is the same at all altitudes.

When ambient (outside) air is drawn into the lungs, it is humidified. Water vapor also has a partial pressure, which turns out to be about 47 torr. The water will displace some of the other gases so their partial pressure will drop. The partial pressure of oxygen in room air is 159 torr, but in the humidified air of the alveolus it is less at about 150 torr. Oxygen is continually removed and carbon dioxide continually added to the gas mixture in the alveoli. Thus the partial pressure of oxygen in the alveolus is only 100. Venous blood has a partial pressure of oxygen of about 40 so the pressure gradient for diffusion is 100 – 40 or 60 mm Hg.

Partial pressures of gases:

GAS	Ambient Air	Alveoli	Arterial blood	Venous blood
pO2	159	100	95	40
pCO2	0.2	40	40	46
pH2O	0.0	47	47	47

pN2	601	573	573	573
TOTAL	760	760	755	706

The Alveolar Gas Equation:

The *Alveolar Gas Equation* allows us to calculate the expected pAO2 (the alveolar oxygen pressure):

$$P_AO_2 = [P_B - PH_2O] \times FiO_2 - (PaCO_2 \times 1.25)$$

Where P_B is atmospheric pressure, PH_2O is the pressure of water vapor, FiO_2 is the fraction of inspired oxygen and the PaCO2 is the arterial carbon dioxide.

For example when the patient is breathing 100% O_2 (the FiO_2 is 1.0) and his or her pCO2 is 40, the pAO2 is:

$$[(760 - 47) \times 1] - (40 \times 1.25) = 663$$

If the patient were on 50% (FiO2 = 0.5) but has a pCO2 of 50, the pAO2 will be:

$$[(760 - 47) \times 0.5] - (50 \times 1.25) = 356.5 - 62.5 \text{ or } 294$$

Lastly, if the patient is on 40% O2 and is in severe respiratory failure with a pCO2 of 80, the pAO2 will be:

$$[(760 - 47) \times 0.4] - (80 \times 1.25) = 285.2 - 100 \text{ or } 185.2$$

Calculating the Alveolar Gas Equation allows us to calculate the A – a O2 gradient which is the gradient or pressure difference between the Alveolar O2 (A) and the arterial O2 (a). The A – a O2 gradient directly influences the rate of diffusion.

IMPORTANT CONCEPTS TO REMEMBER FROM THIS LECTURE

1. Brownian movement is due to:

    The random motion of molecules from an area of high concentration to an area of low concentration

2. The Fio2 is lower on the top of Mount Everest than in Death Valley; true or false:

    False

3. The rate of diffusion is:

    Directly related to the pressure or concentration difference on opposite sides of a semi-permeable membrane and the area available for diffusion. It is inversely related to the thickness of the membrane

4. In normal individuals oxygen is transferred from the blood to the alveolus is:

    One quarter of a second

Chapter Fourteen

Pulmonary Function Testing

The earliest scientist to study lung function was the Greek physician Galan who in the 3rd century had a young man breath in and out of a pig's bladder. He found that the young man's tidal volumes were constant. There stood pulmonary function testing for more than fifteen centuries. Given his apparent lack of interest in pulmonary testing, it is a wonder that Galan's textbooks on medicine were taught in medical schools well into the seventeenth century.

In 1679 the mathematician Giovanni Borelli devised a method of measuring the inspiratory lung volumes. He took a long cylindrical tube and placed one end in a basin of water. He sucked on the open end as deep as he could. He measured the height the water climbed in the tubing. Since he knew the diameter of the tubing he was able to calculate the volume of the fluid in the tube and hence the inspired vital capacity. His estimates however fell short perhaps due to the difference in weight between the water compared to air.

A half century later, the clergyman Stephen Hales, took advantage of Archimedes principles of the displacement of water by air. After a maximal inhalation he blew out all his air into a "bladder". The type of bladder was not specified. He then submerged the filled bladder in a tub of water and determined how much the volume of water rose. He estimated the expired vital capacity at about 3.5 liters, much closer to the truth than Borelli. Boerhaave took Hales one step further. He submerged a man in a tub of water, had him take a deep breath and measured the change in the level of water. That was even more accurate than Hales' bladder! Still the difference in compressibility between water and air probably led to an underestimate of the vital capacity.

In 1831 Charles Thackrah placed an inverted bell jar filled with air into a large basin of water. He then asked his patient to breathe air through a tube that ran from the patient's mouth to the air inside the jar. As the subject blew his air in and out the jar fell and rose with inspiration and expiration. Finally, in 1846, John Hutchinson took Thackrah's device one step further when he developed the water-sealed spirometer which would become the basis of pulmonary studies for more than a century. He also named the subdivisions of lung volume and measured them with his "improved spirometer." He defined the vital capacity as the largest volume that could be exhaled slowly after a maximal inspiration. He studied "members of the fire brigade, metropolitan police, paupers, Thames police, Mixed Class, Grenadier Guards, Royal Horse Guards, Chatham Recruits, Woolrich Marines, Pugilists and Wrestlers, Giants and Dwarfs, Printers, Drayman, Girls, Gentlemen, and Deceased Persons". He studied about 2,130 persons in total and developed tables of predicted values. Pulmonary function testing was finally born. Since then there have been many major advances. In the 1920's, the Collin's spirometer was developed which allowed the measurement of flow rates and in the 1960's, Fry and Hyatt introduced the Flow Volume Curve.

But why do we need pulmonary function testing to start with? There are, of course, several reasons. The first is pragmatic. In Europe during the 17th and 18th century, mining was a major occupation and silicosis was quite common. Many enlightened rulers provided money for workers who became disabled due to mining. This was no doubt due in part so that the ruler could find willing workers to replace the ones who became disabled. Who wanted to be a miner if you knew that in less than ten years you would be disabled unless, of course, you were going to get some compensation? On the other hand, it was easy for a miner to say he was disabled when he really wasn't. Therefore an objective test was needed to determine who deserved some of the ruler's money.

The second reason is to help diagnose lung disease. When someone is short of breath is it due to smoking or is it due to silicosis? Pulmonary testing could help evaluate the cause of the patient's dyspnea. But, with the exception of asthma, a concrete diagnosis can rarely be made with breathing tests alone.

The third reason is to follow the course of a patient's illness. The patient is diagnosed with a pulmonary disease and begun on medication. How do we know if the medication is helping? One way is see if his or her pulmonary testing improves or worsens with therapy.

What do pulmonary function studies (PFTs) actually measure? They measure volumes, flow rates, the rate of diffusion, the compliance, and the patient's response to certain medicines such as albuterol.

Lung Volumes

Lung *volumes* must be separated from lung *capacities*. A volume involves one measurement only. This includes tidal volume (TV), Inspiratory Reserve Volume (IRV), Expiratory Reserve Volume (ERV), and the Residual Volume (RV). The moment we add two or more volumes together we have a capacity. For example, Total Lung Capacity (TLC) is the sum of the IRV + ERV + TV + RV while Functional Residual Capacity is the sum of the RV + ERV, the inspiratory capacity is the sum of the TV + IRV and finally the vital capacity is the sum of the IRV + TV.

Thus we can derive some definitions:

Total Lung Capacity is the total amount of air in the lung after a maximal inspiration.

Vital Capacity is the maximal amount of air that can be exhaled after a maximal inspiration.

Residual Volume is the amount of air left in the lung after a maximal exhalation.

Tidal Volume is the amount of air that moves in and out of the lung during quiet breathing.

Functional Residual Volume is the amount of air left in the lung after a quiet exhalation.

What determines these volumes? Tidal Volume is based on the time constant for the lung and is thus determined by the compliance of the lung and the resistance to air flow. The patient with emphysema breathes deeper and slower than the patient with pulmonary fibrosis.

Total lung capacity is determined by muscle strength in almost all of us. The stronger you are, the greater your lung capacity. For a few people, on the other hand, glottis closure occurs when they take a deep breath and that is what determines their TLC. It is also, of course, determined by the compliance of the lung. If the lung is stiffer than normal, the patient will not be able to exert enough muscle force to expand his or her lungs. If the lung is too compliant, as in a patient with emphysema, the patient can take a deeper breath with the same muscle strength.

Residual Volume is determined solely by muscle strength. Ask someone to exhale fully, and when he or she has totally breathed all the air he or she thought she could breathe out, squeeze them. The extra force of your squeeze will push out even more air. The subject will experience a considerable amount of pain when you do this so chose your subject wisely.

Lastly, Functional Residual Volume is the point at which the tendency of the lung to collapse equals the tendency of the chest wall to expand.

What tests do we do? There are several tests carried out in the standard PFT lab. The first is spirometry, the second the flow-volume curve, the third is the diffusing capacity, and the fourth is the measurement of absolute lung volume. In addition, all laboratories measure the patient's response to a bronchodilator such as albuterol. Research laboratories also measure the lung compliance, the airway resistance, and the methacholine challenge test.

Spirometry:

Spirometry literally means to "measure the breath". The spirometer consists of a large cylindrical bell, closed on top, immersed in a water bath. The patient breathes into one end of a tube while the other end of the tube is inside the bell. As the patient breathes out, the bell rises; as he breathes in the bell falls. The enclosed top of the bell is connected via a pulley to a pen on a rotating drum. As the patient breathes the drum is rotated at a known rate of speed. Thus both volume and time are measured and the flow rates are calculated. Remember: flow is the change in volume with respect to time.

The graph which results is the spirogram. Volume is measured in liters on the Y axis and time is measured in seconds on the X axis. From the graph we can readily make several measurements.

The first measurement is, of course, the vital capacity. From the spirogram, we see immediately the starting volume of the curve, which is, of course, the TLC. We then find the lowest point of the spirogram, which is the residual volume and draw a line from that point, parallel to the X axis, to where it intersects the Y axis. The difference between this volume and the starting volume is the FVC or forced vital capacity. It is a lung volume so it is measured in liters.

We next calculate the FEV1 or the forced expiratory volume in one second. We determine how much air was blown out in the first second. To do that we look on the Y axis to find the starting volume. Then we look at the X axis and draw a line from the 1 second mark straight up to the spirogram. Where the line intersects the spirogram we draw another straight line, parallel to the X axis to where it intersects the Y axis. We measure the change in volume from the starting volume to this second volume. That value is the FEV1, which is the one of the most important measurements used to evaluate a patient's pulmonary status. It is a **lung volume** and is measured in liters.

From these two numbers we calculate one of the most helpful ratios in PFT's, the FEV1/FVC ratio. This ratio is always reduced in patients with obstructive disease. It is always normal, even when the FVC is reduced, in patients with restrictive disease. Never forget that it is also normal in healthy individuals!

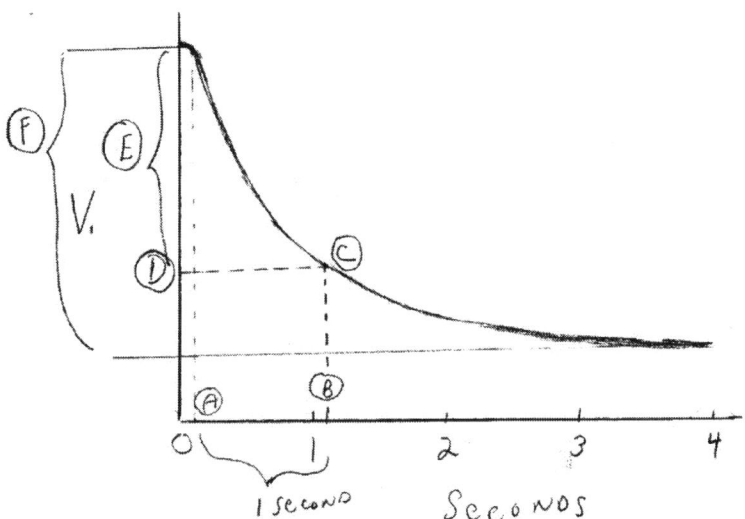

To calculate the FEV1, first find the actual start of the forced expiration which on the graph occurs at point A. Then add one second to that point to give point B. Draw a line from point B parallel to the Y axis. Where it intersects the Spirograph is point C. Draw a line from point C parallel to the X axis. Where it strikes the Y axis is point D. The difference between the volume at the start of the maneuver and point D is the FEV1, which is measured in liters. To get the FEV1/FVC ration divide E by the total vital capacity F. FEV1/FVC = E/F.

The last measurement we can make from the spirogram is the MMF or mid-maximal flow rate. Like the other measurements this is easy to do. Every respiratory therapy student should calculate at least one MMF.

The first step is to divide the vital capacity on the Y axis into four equal parts. The top is the TLC, the first mark down is the lung volume at 75% of the vital capacity, the second mark is the lung volume at 50% of vital capacity, the third mark down is the lung volume at 25%, and the bottom is the lung volume at the residual volume. Next draw a line from the 75% marker, parallel to the X axis till it intersects the spirogram. Then draw a line from this point, parallel to the Y axis till it intersects the X axis. The point is the "time at 75% of the vital capacity". Do the same for the lung volume at 25% of the vital capacity. Then calculate the MMF

MMF = (Volume at 75% - Volume at 25%)/ (time at 75% - time at 25%)

For example if the vital capacity is 4 liters, 75% of the VC is 3 liters, and 25% is 1 liter. Say the time for 75% is 3 seconds and the time for 25% of the VC is 1 second then:

MMF = (3 liters − 1 liter)/ (3 seconds - 1 second)

2/2 = 1 <u>liter per second</u>

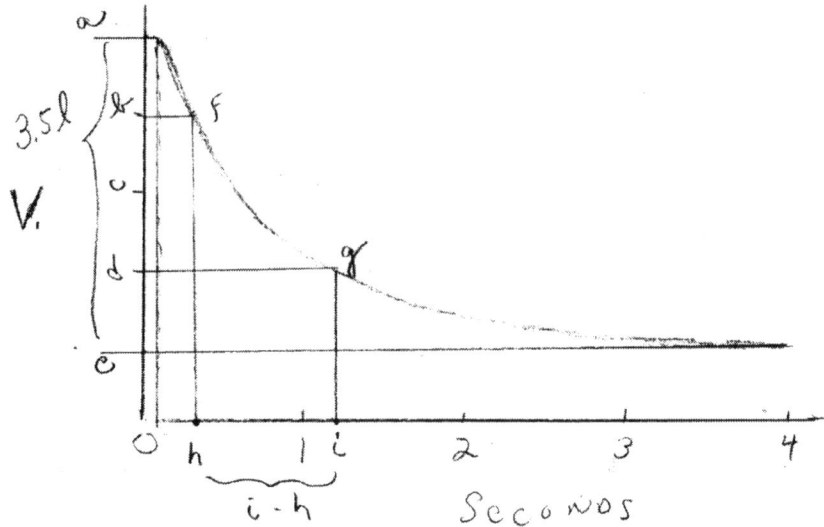

To calculate the MMF, first measure the Forced Vital Capacity on the Y axis and divide it into four equal parts. On the graph: a = TLC, b = 75% of the VC, c = 50% of the VC, d = 25% of the VC, and e = the RV.

Next, draw lines from 25% and 75% of VC (points d and b) parallel to the X axis to where they intersect the Spirograph. These points are g and f. Then construct lines from f and g parallel to the Y axis till where they intersect the X axis. These are points i and h respectively.

The MMF = (d – b)/(i – h) or 1.8 liters/1 second or 1.8 liters/sec.

Note that the FEV1 is a lung volume measured in liters while the MMF is a flow rate measured in liters/second.

Simple spirometry using the Collin's spirometer is rarely used today, but the measurements it generates are still the most important measurements in the armament of the respiratory therapist.

The FEV1 looks directly at large airway function as well as muscle strength. It is the best predictor of how a patient will do with surgery. The MMF looks at small airways function but it has such a wide range of normal values that it is not as helpful as the FEV1.

Flow-Volume Loop:

Most respiratory therapists will do PFTs using newer machines that produce the "flow-volume loop". The flow-volume loop eliminates time from the measurement. Instead of volume versus time, we have volume versus flow. Flow is on the Y axis and volume is on the X axis. Inspiration is below the volume line; exhalation is above the volume line.

What can we measure from the flow volume loop? Looking at the curve, we can immediately see the "peak expiratory flow rate" which is the maximal rate of flow the patient can exhale. We can also pick a volume on the X axis, say 50%, and by drawing a line perpendicular to the X axis to where it intersects the curve calculate the flow rate at that particular volume which would be flow at 50% of the vital capacity or V50.

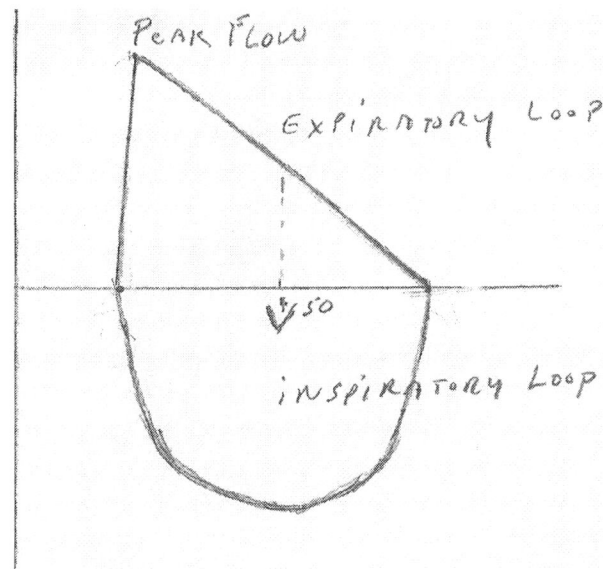

Flow Volume Curve: Below the volume line is inspiratory flow; above the line is expiratory flow. The peak flow is readily seen as is the flow at 50% of the vital capacity. But there is no FEV1 or MMF to be seen.

But we can't measure the FEV1 or the MMF from the flow volume curve! The machine must calculate those values for you.

The flow-volume loop is more helpful in understanding pulmonary mechanics than in the diagnosis of disease. We still use the FEV1 and MMF but the flow-volume curve can tell us more about physiology. The first part of the curve, near the start of exhalation, looks at large airway function, just like the FEV1, while the middle and lower portion of the curve looks at small airways disease. In young people the curve is a straight line from its peak to its lowest point at RV. But in older patients and especially in patients with chronic obstructive disease, it is "scooped out". The curve falls off rapidly from its peak. This suggests, that the large airways are intact, while the smaller and collapsible airways are narrowed by the force exhalation exerts on the pleural pressure. The small airways are compressed by the increased pleural pressures of a forced exhalation.

An interesting study the student can do is to have a fellow student exhale maximally from TLC with ever increasing force while measuring the subject's exhalation flow-volume curve. At first the patient's expiratory flow-volume curve is low and flat. As the force increases, the part of the curve near the start of exhalation increases, but it soon becomes apparent that the middle and end part of the flow-volume loop have a maximum value. Thus the early part of the curve, near total lung capacity, depends solely upon the effort the subject exerts. The harder he or she exerts, the greater the flow rate. On the other hand, the middle and end part of the curve are totally dependent on the airway itself. The early part of the flow-volume curve is called "effort dependent"; the middle and end of the curve are called "airway dependent".

Absolute Lung Volumes:

The actual measurement of lung volumes, especially total lung capacity, the residual volume, and the functional residual capacity are more complex.

The total lung capacity can actually be measured accurately from a standard chest radiograph but the work requires hours to do and is thus not very practical.

Rather we measure the TLC, RV, and FRC by taking advantage of either Boyle's law or the Ideal Gas Law: $PV = nRT$, where n is the moles of the gas, R is the gas constant, and T is the temperature. Boyle's law is used in both the Nitrogen Wash-out and Helium Wash-in while the Ideal Gas Law is used in the "body box" or body plethysmography.

Using Boyle's law, in a closed system, Volume Times the Concentration is Constant

$$V1 \times C1 = V2 \times C2$$

Where V1 and C1 are the volume of the system and concentration of the gas at the start of the procedure and V2 and C2 are the system volume and gas concentration at the end.

Thus, if we know C1, V2, and C2, we can calculate V1. The most commonly used test is the Helium Wash-in. The Helium Wash-in is done in two steps utilizing a closed system which contains a port for the administration of Helium, a spirometer, a device for removing carbon dioxide in order to prevent a build-up of the gas in the closed system, and a second device for adding oxygen to keep the volume constant as well as a port for the patient to breathe into.

The first step is to add a measured amount of Helium to the closed system before the patient is connected. Time is allowed for the Helium to diffuse throughout the system and the Helium concentration in the system is measured. The volume of the system is measured using Boyle's law.

In the second stage, the patient is connected to the system and allowed to breathe till the Helium concentration becomes constant. While he breathes he produces carbon dioxide which must be removed. The patient also consumes oxygen. To keep the volume of the system constant oxygen needs to be added. From the final Helium concentration the volume of the total system (patient and circuitry is determined). The volume of the circuitry is then subtracted to get the patient's volume.

The nitrogen wash-out system is simpler. Our lungs have 78% nitrogen. Thus, if a patient breathes in 100% oxygen and we collect all the exhaled gas, all the nitrogen in the collected gas will have come from the patient. Thus we know the starting concentration of nitrogen, and we measure the final concentration of nitrogen and the total expired volume of gas which is V2.

$$V1 = (N2 \times V2)/N1$$

N1 is the nitrogen concentration in the patient, V1 is the volume of the patient, N2 is the final nitrogen concentration we collected which was exhaled by the patient and V2 is the total volume exhaled and collected from the patient. Thus we measure N2 and V2. We know that N1 = .78 and we calculate V1 from the equation.

The Nitrogen wash-out has some shortcomings. We don't know for certain exactly where the patient was in his vital capacity when we began the test. He could have been at FRC but he could have been at TLC. We don't know. We thus have a "turn-in error". In addition the blood has nitrogen. Some of the blood N2 will be washed into the lungs and become part of our measured N2. We must guess-estimate this amount based on how long the study took to perform.

While the Helium wash-in avoids both these errors. However, both the nitrogen and helium test can't measure areas of the lung with a long time-constant such as large bullae. Both tests underestimate the lung volume in patients with cysts or large blebs.

The body plethysmography uses the Ideal Gas Law, PV = nRT, where nRT is a constant. Thus, just as in Boyle's law, in a closed box P1 X V1 must equal P2 X V2. Simply, the patient is placed in a box of known volume. The patient breathes quietly into a mouthpiece which has a shutter. At some point the shutter is closed, the patient pants, and the change in volume and change in pressure inside the box are measured during the panting. The volume of the subject at the start is equal to the pressure of the subject divided by the ratio of the change in pressure to the change in volume. While the mathematics is complex, the results are excellent. The body box will measure the volume of cysts and blebs in the lungs which neither gas study does well. The only problem is that if the patient has drunk a lot of bubbly water before the test, the gas in the stomach will also be measured.

Diffusing Capacity:

Diffusion is measured using carbon monoxide (CO)! Why carbon monoxide? It sounds dangerous to me.

Remember the Fick equation as applied to the lung:

Rate of diffusion = [K X (Palv – Prbc) X Area]/thickness of the membrane

(Palv is the alveolar pressure of the gas; Prbc is the "back pressure" in the red blood cell; K is the constant of diffusion)

Oxygen could be used to measure the rate of diffusion but oxygen has a problem. While the red blood cells take up oxygen voraciously, there is a definite back pressure. The alveolar oxygen level is 100 torr and the venous oxygen level is about 40 torr. Thus the pressure gradient is 100 – 40 or 60 torr. **However, we can't measure the actual back pressure!** We have to estimate it! On the other hand, carbon monoxide is taken up even more voraciously than oxygen (210 times more in fact) and there thus, with few exceptions, there is never a back pressure. We can ignore the back pressure completely with few exceptions (tobacco smokers and patients with anemia). The Fick equation then becomes:

Rate of diffusion = [K X Palv X Area]/thickness

When we use carbon monoxide all we have to do is know how much carbon monoxide we give the patient at the start of the test and how much is left at the end. From that we can determine how much gas was taken up over what time. We also measure the lung volume at the same time so we can compare the rate of diffusion to the lung volume at which it was measured.

Most of the time a single breath diffusing capacity is performed. The patient inhales a given amount of a gas containing carbon monoxide. He holds his breathe for ten seconds. When he exhales the carbon monoxide is measured. The difference between the carbon monoxide at the beginning and end of the breath hold is calculated and then divided by the number of seconds the patient held his breath. That is the diffusing capacity. Of course, in real life the equations used by the computers in PFT equipment are more than two pages long. Thank heavens for computers.

Normal Values:

Lung volumes and diffusion are directly related to sex, age, height and race. In general, men have greater values for lung volumes and diffusion as do tall people. As we age, these values all decrease.

Race plays a big role as well. Blacks have a 12% lower TLC, FEV1, and FVC as well as a 7% lower FRC and RV. Asian Americans have a 6% lower TLC, FEV1, FVC, FRC, and RV. The corrections do not apply to the RV/TLC or FEV1/FVC ratios.

When reporting test results you must specify whether or not you "race corrected" them. The most commonly used table of normal values is Morris, et al. The values were obtained from Mormons who don't smoke or drink so they are as representative of what is truly normal as normal can be. However, they are not race-corrected.

Diffusion has its own problems. Smoking, especially cigars, can affect the diffusing capacity by causing a "back pressure". We noted that in normal subjects there is no back pressure but in cigar smokers the carbon monoxide in the blood can be quite high resulting in a significant back pressure.

There are some other situations we need to be aware of. If we find a decreased diffusion with normal spirometry we need to think about anemia, pulmonary vascular disorders such as pulmonary emboli and pulmonary artery disease, as well as patients with very early emphysema or interstitial lung disease. If we have a patient with restrictive lung disease but normal diffusion we need to think about neuromuscular disease as well as diseases of the chest wall. Finally if we have a very high diffusing capacity we should think about asthma, obesity, or bleeding into the lungs (intrapulmonary hemorrhage).

Effects of medications:

Asthma is probably the only disease that can be firmly diagnosed in the pulmonary function laboratory. Moreover, the diagnosis is fairly straightforward. When a patient is seen with suspected asthma, if his spirometry is abnormal, give him a bronchodilator such as a beta-adrenergic agent like albuterol to inhale. If his FEV1 increases 12%, he has asthma or, less likely, an asthmatic form of chronic bronchitis. On the other hand, if his baseline spirometry is normal, give him tiny, tiny inhalations of a medicine which causes bronchoconstriction such as Methacholine which is an acetyl choline analog. If his FEV1 decreases 20% at very low doses of the agent, the patient very likely has asthma. The methacholine challenge testing is 95% sensitive and 95% specific. It is the most accurate test available to diagnosis asthma.

Airway Resistance

The measurement of airway resistance (Raw) is more difficult and is generally done in specialized laboratories or research laboratories. The most common approach is to use an oscillator, which is basically a "speaker" which sends small air waves into the airway during quiet breathing. The small changes in pressure and airflow due to the tiny waves are measured and the resistance (pressure/air flow) is calculated. The test is simple to perform and is done during quiet tidal volume breathing so the patient does not need to be able to perform complex maneuvers such as a vital capacity. It can even be done in young children who find it difficult to do the standard pulmonary testing.

The airway resistance can also be measured using the whole body plethysmograph by suddenly stopping air flow with a shutter while the patient is panting and measuring the immediate changes in pressure and volume. From complex graphics the Raw as well as conductance (inverse of resistance) can be calculated.

One of the advantages to using the "speaker" system is that the resistance can be measured while the patient inhales and exhales. Thus, the relationship between resistance and lung volume can be evaluated.

Putting it all together:

PFTs allow us to get a handle on the pulmonary causes of shortness of breath. We can use the PFT to readily distinguish between obstructive and restrictive disease:

Obstructive Disease is characterized by:

1. The flow rate is **reduced out of proportion** to change in volume
2. The RV/TLC ratio is increased
3. The FEV1/FVC ratio is always decreased

Restrictive Disease is characterized by:

1. The reduction in lung volumes with relative preservation of flow rates. Flow rates and lung volumes are reduced proportionately.

We can further evaluate the types of restrictive disease. In general, in the patient with restrictive disease, the TLC, FRC, and RV are all reduced but in the patient with chest wall disease causing restriction, such as kyphoscoliosis, the RV may be increased while the TLC and FRC are decreased. Moreover if the restriction is due to muscle weakness as in a patient with a neurological problem such as Guillain-Barre or Myasthenia gravis, the FRC IS NORMAL but the TLC is decreased and the RV increased. Finally in a patient with obesity the TLC and RV are normal but the FRC is decreased due to the chest wall mass.

Most importantly, in patients with musculoskeletal disease, regardless of the cause, the diffusion capacity is normal while in patients with obesity the diffusing capacity is usually increased though in a few it is normal or decreased.

The following graph should be tattooed on the respiratory therapist's chest.

	Obstructive disease		Restrictive disease	
Test	**Asthma/bronchitis**	**emphysema**	**lung disease**	**chest wall**
FVC	decreased	decreased	decreased	decreased
FEV1	decreased **out of proportion** to lung volume		decreased **in proportion** to lung volume	
TLC	increased	increased	decreased	decreased
DCO	normal	**decreased**	**decreased**	normal

IMPORTANT CONCEPTS TO REMEMBER FROM THIS LECTURE

1. Spirometry relates:

    Volume to time

2. The Nitrogen Washout takes advantage of:

    Boyle's law

3. If a person has a low diffusing capacity but otherwise his studies are normal he or she might have:

    Vascular disease, anemia, neuromuscular disease, early emphysema, or early pulmonary fibrosis

4. The flow volume curve eliminates:

    Time

5. The Morris table of normal values was calculated in:

    Mormons who neither smoke nor drink

Lecture Fifteen

Control of Ventilation

We must address two different concepts. The first concept is that although the lung does not have any sensory nerves for detecting pain nor does it have motor nerves of the type found in the large muscles of the legs and arms, it is innervated by a complex of nerves that make up the autonomic nervous system. We might call the autonomic nervous system the "automatic nervous system" because we are totally unaware of what the nervous system is doing. It does its job without us making a conscious decision. We don't tell our airways to dilate or constrict but they do it when they need to. When we have to cough in order to clear out an irritant that entered our air passage, we automatically take a deep breath, the bronchi constrict, and then we cough it out.

The second concept is that, like our bronchial tubes, our frequency and depth of breathing is automatic. When we decide we are going to go for a run, our rate and depth of breathing increase, even before we take our first step.

How do these things happen?

We will examine the control of ventilation in two parts: the autonomic nervous system of the lung and the central nervous system control of ventilation.

Autonomic Nervous System:

The autonomic nervous system consists of two parts, the sympathetic nervous system and the parasympathetic nervous system. We are all familiar with the "flight or fight", adrenaline driven, sympathetic nervous system. Some of us are probably just as familiar with the "Let's chill out at the barbecue", acetyl choline driven, parasympathetic system.

The sympathetic nervous system stimulates the heart to beat faster and, as we noted many lectures ago, increases the contractility of the heart as well as raises the blood pressure. It also increases the blood flow to the brain and the muscles needed to fight or flee. In the lungs the adrenergic system is a bronchodilator, which makes sense. After all, if you are going to flee you want to be able to move as much air as possible in and out of your lungs. On the other hand, blood flow to the kidneys and gut is reduced.

Adrenaline is released from nerve endings of the sympathetic nervous system. In the lung the adrenaline converts adenosine triphosphate (remember our very first lecture) into cyclic adenosine-monophosphate which causes bronchodilation.

The parasympathetic nervous system is more concerned with digestion, urination, and sex. The parasympathetic system is responsible for stimulation of "rest-and-digest" or "feed and breed" activities that occur when the body is at rest, especially after eating a good meal. These functions include sexual arousal, salivation, formation of tears, urination, digestion as well as defecation. It increases blood flow to the mesenteric arteries making the gut work better. It also slows the heart and it narrows the bronchial tubes. One of the most important parasympathetic nerves is the Vagus

Nerve. The Latin word vagus means "wandering". The Vagus Nerve innervates the lungs, heart, and gut. Even the Recurrent Laryngeal Nerve, which actually passes through the left upper thorax around what remains of the Ductus Arteriosus in order to innervate the left vocal cord of the larynx, originates from the Vagus Nerve. It truly wanders! The parasympathetic nervous system secretes acetyl choline which attaches to the muscarinic receptors found on endothelial cells. Activation of the receptors causes the conversion of guanosine triphosphate into cyclic guanosine-monophosphate which then causes the smooth muscle of the airways to contract resulting in bronchoconstriction.

The parasympathetic nervous system is involved in the "cough reflex". There are exquisitely sensitive sensory fibers located on the posterior wall of the trachea, the carina and the posterior walls of the large bronchi. The lightest touch will activate the receptors which then send a signal via the vagus nerve to the medulla which then sends efferent signals to diaphragm via the phrenic nerve, the intercostal muscles via the intercostal nerves, the larynx via the vagus nerve, and the abdominal muscles via the spinal nerves. A complex dance ensues. The diaphragm and external intercostal muscles contract, creating a large negative intrapleural pressure around the lung. Air rushes into the lungs in order to equalize the pressure. Next the glottis slams shut closing the airway. Following this the abdominal muscles contract and the diaphragm relaxes. Simultaneously all the expiratory muscles contract increasing the pressure of air within the lungs. Then the vocal cords relax opening the glottis releasing air at over 100 mph. The bronchi and non-cartilaginous portions of the trachea contract which clears out any irritants attached to the respiratory lining.

Respiratory Centers in the Brain

Breathing is totally automatic. We just don't walk around saying to ourselves, "breathe in; breathe out." We just breathe. In addition, we must inhale and then have a controlled exhalation when we talk. When we cough we don't say, "Take a deep breath, close the glottis, contract all the muscles of exhalation, open the glottis." We just cough. When we jog we don't give our body instructions about how fast and how deep we should breathe. We just concentrate on where we are putting our feet. When we sing or play the clarinet or flute, no matter how complex the music, we do it. No instruction is needed, although I must admit, practice is definitely of value.

It is clear that a very complex system is required in order to accomplish all these tasks. This system requires several parts of the brain, several nerves both sensory and motor, as well as the muscles of the abdomen and chest wall in order to function.

These systems must be integrated silently without our control. But we must be able to tell ourselves to take a deep breath or to cough whenever we want. Thus cerebral cortex must have the ability to override the functioning of the "automatic centers".

The brain is quite complex. It is made up of many parts. The large bulbous part at the top is the cerebral cortex. The "gray" cells of the cerebral cortex have areas for controlling our emotions in the prefrontal cortex, an area for sensation and a motor area in the mid portion and an area for vision in the posterior portion. Just below and posterior to the cerebral cortex is the cerebellum which is responsible for coordinating our movements so that we don't fall when we walk, so that our speech is fluid and so that our singing is harmonious.

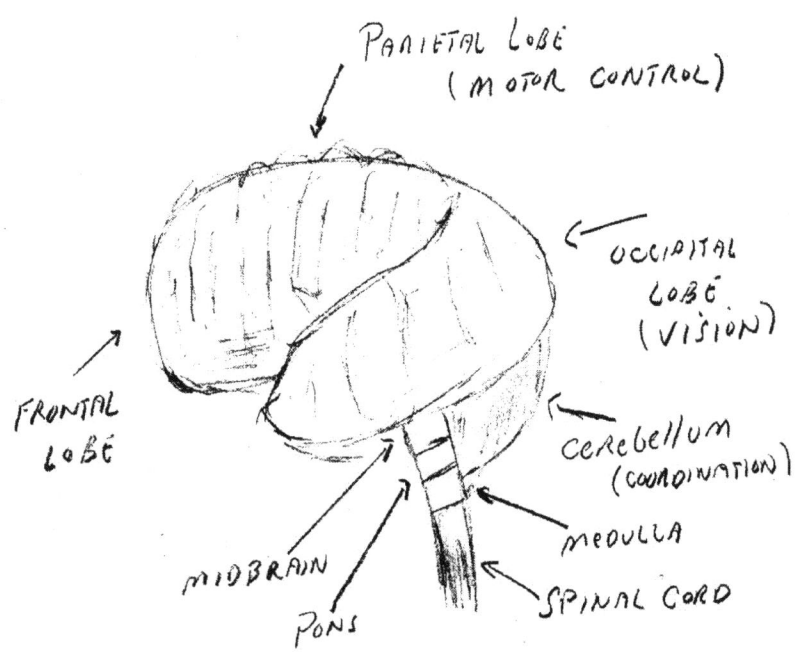

Below the cerebral cortex is the brainstem, the most primitive part of the brain. It consists of several organs. The hippocampus, responsible for memory (London cabdrivers have enormous hippocampi), the mid brain, the pons, and the lowest part of the brain, the medulla.

The pons and the medulla contain the respiratory centers. These are the centers that control how fast and how deep we breathe.

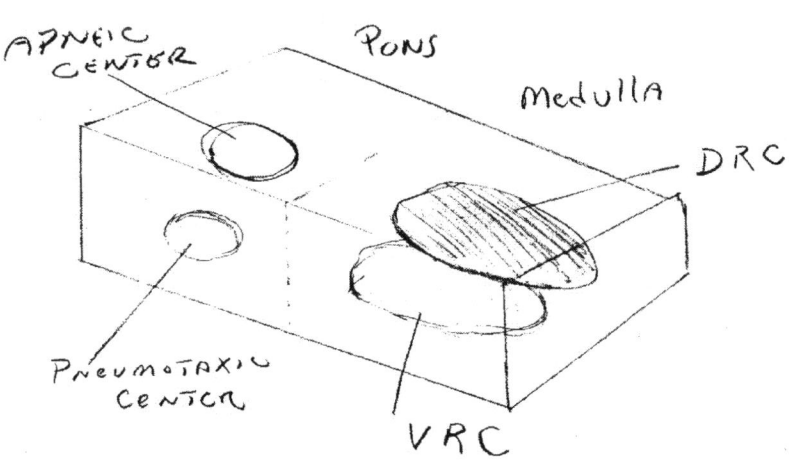

The medulla has two centers, a *ventral respiratory center* (VRC) and a *dorsal respiratory center* (DRC). The DRC functions as a gatekeeper. It takes in information from stretch receptors in the lung as well as chemoreceptors and baroreceptors in the aortic and carotid bodies and chemoreceptors in the medulla itself. It also is fed information from the cerebral cortex. It organizes the information which it then passes its conclusions to the VRC. The VRC controls both inspiration and expiration. It coordinates the rate and depth of breathing. It has two parts. One part of the VRC stimulates inspiration via the phrenic and intercostal nerves while one part of the VRC turns off inspiration.

The Pons is located directly above the Medulla and below the Midbrain. The Pontine Centers modify and fine tune the VRC.

Like the medulla the Pons also contains two respiratory centers. The first is the Pneumotaxic Center (Pontine Respiratory Group) which smooths out the transition from inspiration to expiration and expiration to inspiration. The second is the Apneustic (Apneic) Center. When it is activated it causes a long, held breath. This long breath is inhibited by the Pneumotaxic Center and the Herring-Breuer Reflex which is the lung inflation reflex.

Neurologic input into the medulla comes from multiple sources including receptors in the brain, systemic chemoreceptors found in blood vessels, baroreceptors, stretch or "J" receptors found in the lung and the cerebral cortex.

The central chemoreceptors are found in the medulla directly exposed to the cerebrospinal fluid (CSF). They respond to H^+ ions. Carbon dioxide readily crosses the blood brain barrier, whereas H^+ ions do not. But when CO_2 enters the brain it combines with water to produce H^+ ions and HCO_3^-. The H^+ ions stimulate the medullary centers to increase ventilation.

Peripheral chemoreceptors are found in the aortic and carotid bodies. The receptor cells are in direct communication with the blood. <u>They are activated when the **PaO_2** drops below 60 but are inactivated when it drops below 30.</u> Thus the response to severe hypoxemia is depressed. **The cells do NOT respond to SaO_2 however.** Stimulation of the peripheral receptors causes the heart to beat faster and increases both the systemic and pulmonary resistance.

In a patient with chronic obstructive lung disease who has had CO_2 retention for some time, more blood borne HCO_3^- will slowly cross into the CSF and combine with the H^+ ions raising the pH back towards normal. The central nervous system stimulus for hyperventilation will subside, leaving only the peripheral receptors response to PaO_2 intact. If a patient with chronic CO_2 retention who has blood gases which show a PaO_2 of 40, a $PaCO_2 = 80$ and a pH = 7.40 is given high flow oxygen increasing his PaO_2 to more than 60, he will stop breathing because he will have lost both his central and peripheral drive to breath.

The peripheral chemoreceptors are also stimulated by decreased pH, especially when not due to increased $PaCO_2$. This may occur in shock, when lactic acid accumulates, or diabetic coma, when ketones accumulate, or renal failure, when sulphates and phosphates increase. In addition, fever, nicotine, hypoperfusion and even increased $PaCO_2$ will stimulate the peripheral receptors. The response of the peripheral chemoreceptor to $PaCO_2$ is faster than the response of the central receptors but is much weaker.

Two other factors are important in the regulation of ventilation. We all know that when we get excited or emotional we breathe faster and deeper. This is due to the part of the brain called the Hypothalamus. Lastly we can control our breathing. We can decide to hold our breath or we can decide to hyperventilate. Thus signals from the cerebral cortex can override the automatic functions of the respiratory system.

The nerves involved in the input and output of the respiratory center are extensive. The Glossopharyngeal Nerve is the 9th cranial nerve. It arises from the medulla and has sensory fibers from the pharynx, carotid body and carotid sinus. It is also important in swallowing. After all we don't want to breathe and swallow at the same time.

The Vagus Nerve is the 10th cranial nerve. It has both sensory and motor neurons. It is important in the irritant reaction of the airways and it transmits data from the stretch receptors in the lung. In addition to these sensory functions, it also has motor fibers which cause a slowing of the heart and bronchoconstriction. It is also important in the Herring-Breuer reflex described below.

Motor output from the medulla is carried not only by the Vagus Nerve but also by the Phrenic Nerve which originates from C3-C5 nerve roots and carries motor fibers to the diaphragm and the thoracic and abdominal motor neurons to the intercostal and abdominal muscles.

There are several reflexes which we need to be aware of:

1. **Herring-Breuer Reflex**

    When the stretch (J) receptors in the pleura and bronchi become stimulated by lung over-inflation, a signal is sent to the respiratory centers to stop inspiration. This reflex is mediated by the Vagus nerve.

2. **Deflation Reflex**

    Compression of the lung stimulates an increased rate of breathing

3. **Irritant Reflex**

    Noxious gases and mucus stimulate receptors in the trachea and bronchi which via the vagus nerve cause increased respiration, cough, sneezing and narrowing of the bronchial tubes.

4. **J-fiber or Juxtapulmonary-Capillary Receptors**

    In addition to their response to over-inflation, J receptors also respond to some chemicals including serotonin and bradykinin as well as mechanical stimulation such as alveolar inflammation, lung deflation and pulmonary emboli. Stimulation of the J receptors causes a rapid, shallow breathing pattern

5. **Peripheral Proprioceptor Reflexes**

    There are also Proprioceptors which sense movement located in the muscles and tendons. When we start to walk or run, the proprioceptors send signals to the medulla sow we will breathe faster.

6. **Pain Receptor Reflexes**

>Lastly there are pain receptors found in the muscles and skin, which send signals to the medulla to increase respiration. **Sudden pain or sudden cold exposure causes a short episode of apnea; more chronic pain causes hyperventilation**

There are numerous neurological diseases that can directly affect the control of respiration. The most common include narcotic drug overdose which slows respiration by depressing the respiratory centers in the medulla. Chronic brainstem strokes and Multiple Sclerosis (MS) can also damage the cells in the respiratory centers.

Both multiple brainstem strokes and Multiple Sclerosis can damage the brainstem making it impossible to swallow without choking. A stroke is caused by a blockage in a blood vessel to part of the brain which then dies. Multiple sclerosis involves the destruction of the myelin sheath which is responsible for providing nutrition to the central nervous system neurons.

Other neurologic diseases can interfere with the muscles of respiration. These include Muscular Dystrophy, Guillain-Barre or ascending paralysis, Myasthenia Gravis, and trauma to the spinal cord.

Lecture Notes: Anatomy and Physiology for the Respiratory Therapist

IMPORTANT CONCEPTS TO REMEMBER FROM THIS LECTURE

1. The Medulla has two respiratory centers; what are they and what do they do?

    The ventral respiratory center controls both inspiration and expiration

    The dorsal respiratory center assimilates data from the peripheral stretch receptors and chemoreceptors and sends the information to the ventral respiratory center

2. The Herring-Breuer reflex is:

    The cessation of inspiration caused by the medullary respiratory center (VRC) when the lung is overinflated.

3. The peripheral receptors respond to:

    Only the pO2, **NOT the O2 content**. A low O2 content due to anemia or carbon monoxide poisoning will **not** stimulate the peripheral receptors.

4. The peripheral chemoreceptors are activated when the paO2 is:

    Less than 60

5. The peripheral chemoreceptors are inactivated when the paO2 is:

    Less than 30

Peter A. Petroff, MD

Lecture Sixteen

Overview of Obstructive Lung Disorders.

Obstructive diseases are diseases of the airways or their supporting structure. They are characterized by a decrease in expiratory airflow out of proportion to a decrease in lung volumes. In other words, pulmonary function testing shows a decreased vital capacity and FEV1 in both obstructive and restrictive lung disease but in obstructive lung disease the FEV1 is reduced OUT OF PROPORTION to the decrease in the vital capacity. The ratio between the FEV1 and the FVC is reduced.

The *Global Obstructive Lung Disease Initiative* or GOLD defines chronic obstructive lung disease:

"COPD is a disease state characterized by airflow limitation which is not fully reversible."

The researchers also state that the airflow limitation is progressive and is associated with an *inflammatory response*. In other words, **COPD is an inflammatory disease of the small airways with lung destruction and subepithelial fibrosis and squamous metaplasia.**

The FEV1 correlates with the thickness of the small airway wall.

Obstructive lung disease can be divided into four groups:

1. Emphysema due to loss of elastic supporting structure.
2. Chronic bronchitis due to inflammation of the airways.
3. Chronic Asthma characterized by only partially reversibility.
4. Bronchiectasis characterized by destruction of the bronchioles.

For the most part when we speak about COPD we generally are referring to emphysema, chronic bronchitis, and bronchiectasis. Asthma, which is potentially completely reversible, is generally not included in COPD but is treated separately.

COPD is the fourth leading cause of death worldwide. In our country 120,000 die of the disease every year, one death every four minutes. There are more than 15 million Americans with the disease and the disease is now more common in women than in men.

COPD, whether it be emphysema, chronic bronchitis, chronic asthma, or bronchiectasis, is always characterized by inflammation. There is an increase in cells associated with inflammation including the neutrophils, alveolar macrophages and the T8 or "killer" lymphocytes. There is an increase in toxic chemicals such as peroxidase and nitric oxide, both of which cause cell death. The neutrophils and macrophages also activate the proteinases, chemicals that causes destruction of the alveolar walls. The inflammatory response narrows the airways and results in destruction of the supporting structure of the lung as well as the alveoli and capillaries.

These changes result in characteristic physiological findings. The forced expiratory vital capacity is reduced and, with the exception of asthma, does not respond or responds minimally to B adrenergic agents such as Albuterol. On the other hand because of the loss of supporting tissue, the total lung capacity (TLC) and residual volume (RV) are both increased and the ratio between the RV and the TLC (the RV/TLC ratio) is increased even more. Lastly, in patients with emphysema, the diffusion capacity is decreased because of the loss of alveoli and capillaries.

The two most common types of COPD are emphysema and chronic bronchitis. The patient with emphysema is often described as the "Pink Puffer". The patient with emphysema has shortness of breath as his main concern. If he doesn't smoke he won't even cough. His blood gases are NORMAL. They look exactly like yours and mine. His oxygen level is normal as is pH and carbon dioxide. However, his chest radiograph will show hyperinflation and he will appear barrel chested. His accessory muscles of respiration will be prominent. When he sits, he will sit in the "tripod position" with his elbow resting on the arms of his chair or on your desk. Since his disease is due to the permanent destruction of the alveolar walls and capillaries, when he develops cor pulmonale, there is no treatment, and he will die within six months.

On the other hand the patient with chronic bronchitis is described as the "Blue Bloater". He complains bitterly about his cough and phlegm but is short of breath only when he exerts himself, which is infrequent. At rest he is relaxed, bloated, and blue due to his low oxygen level. He is a member of the "50 50 50 Club." His pO_2 is 50, his pCO_2 is 50 and his hematocrit is 50. The hematocrit should be less than 45 but with the patient's low oxygen level, his kidneys pump out more erythropoietin which makes bone marrow pump out more red blood cells. The "Blue Bloater" also gets cor pulmonale, but in his case, it is due to the hypoxia often associated with an infection. Treating the infection and correcting the hypoxia improves the cor pulmonale, so he goes in out of cor pulmonale frequently. The episodes of cor pulmonale may, in fact, go on for several years.

Emphysema

Emphysema is due to the destruction of the elastic supporting structures of the lung and the alveolar capillary membranes. The airway obstruction is due to both narrowing of the small airways due to inflammation as well as to the collapse of these airways during exhalation due to the loss of the elastic supporting structure.

Smoking is certainly the most frequent cause of emphysema. But the disease can also be caused by the inhalation of cocaine, which damages the small blood vessels of the lung. Cocaine can also cause heart attacks and strokes. Cadmium can also cause emphysema. People who had a low birth weight or who had recurrent childhood infections can develop the disease as well. Sarcoidosis, a restrictive lung disorder we will encounter in the next lecture, can also cause emphysema. Emphysema is also more common in people with allergy (atopy) and people who have type A blood. A lifetime of poorly controlled asthma can also result in emphysema. A recent study (Raju, S. et. al, Am J. Resp. and Crit. Care Medicine, November 2.2018) showed that poor rural areas had the highest rates of COPD. For every unit decrease in household income in a rural setting, the incidence of COPD increased 8%. More importantly, if a household used coal for heating, there was a 9% increased risk of COPD. Lastly, emphysema is also a hereditary disease. People who are deficient in Alpha 1 Antitrypsin may develop emphysema.

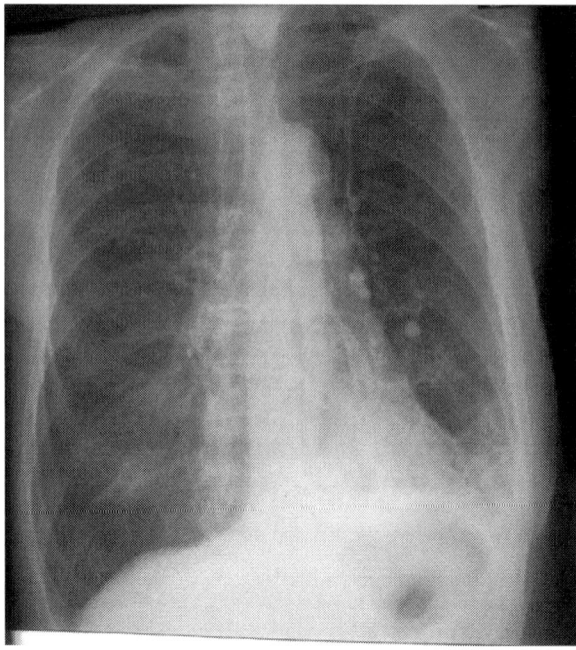

The typical chest x-ray of a patient with emphysema shows hyperinflation. The right lung shows marked widening of the ribs spaces and a flattened diaphragm. The changes are not seen on the left because of loss of volume due to left lower lobe atelectasis. The tiny nodule in the left mid lung field may be a cancer.

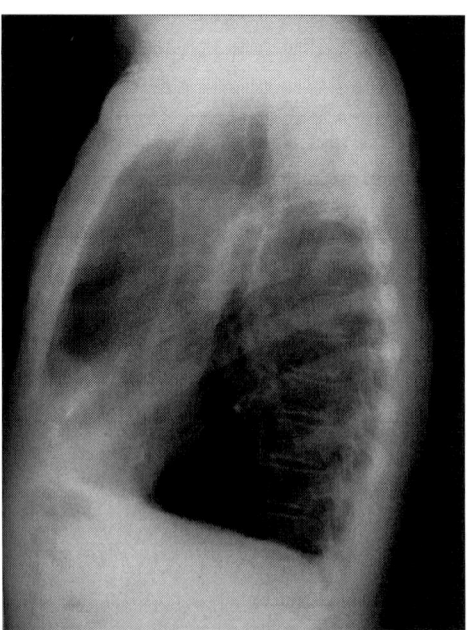

The lateral chest x-ray shows marked flattening of the diaphragm. Even more interesting is that the vertebral column is severely osteoporotic. Osteoporosis is often found in patients with emphysema. This patient also has a pacemaker.

The diagnosis of emphysema is a pathologic diagnosis not a clinical diagnosis. In the past, the only way to be sure the patient had emphysema was to do an autopsy. Now, because of the high resolution CAT scan of the chest (HRCT), the diagnosis can readily be made while the patient is still alive. The HRCT will show the bullae and blebs diagnostic of the disease.

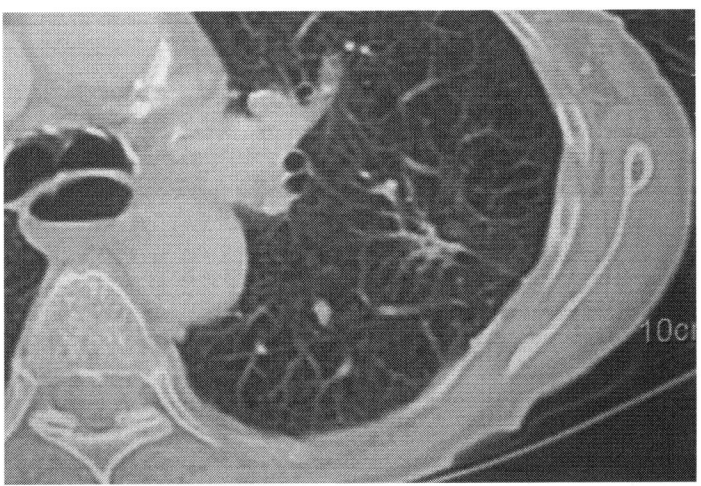

The typical HRCT of the patient with emphysema. The trachea is on the left hand side of the x-ray with the esophagus and vertebral column directly behind. To the right of the vertebral column is the aorta, with a calcified plaque in its lateral wall. The lung shows numerous tiny blebs and a few large bullae. The linear structures are blood vessels.

Emphysema is divided into two large types: centrilobular, and panlobular. Centrilobular involves mainly the respiratory bronchioles while panlobular involves the entire acinar structure as well including the respiratory bronchioles, alveolar ducts and alveolar sacs. There is often inflammation of the small airways associated with centrilobular emphysema. In panlobular emphysema there is no fibrosis or scar tissue visible. While the disease is an inflammatory disease, fibrosis is not present.

Centrilobular emphysema is most often due to smoking and is associated with chronic bronchitis. Panlobular disease is often hereditary. The most classic example of panlobular emphysema is Alpha 1 Antitrypsin deficiency.

We must take a brief aside into the study of genetics. Each of us has 23 pairs of autosomal chromosomes, responsible for things like hair and eye color, and one pair of sex chromosomes either a pair of X's if you are a young lady or an X and a Y if you are a young man. One of the pair of genes comes from our father; one of the pair of genes comes from our mother.

There are about 20,000 genes for coding proteins found on our chromosomes. Each pair of genes is made up of two *alleles*. Some of these alleles can have hundreds of variations as we will see when we look into cystic fibrosis. The *genotype* of a person is the gene makeup. The *phenotype* is how the effects of the gene look to us.

An allele can either be *dominant* which means that if it is one of the pair of alleles, it will determine the phenotype. The allele can also be codominant meaning that each gene in the pair contributes to the phenotype. Lastly, the allele can be recessive, meaning that both alleles must be present in order to be expressed as the phenotype.

If both alleles are the same, the person is homozygote for the gene. If the alleles are different the person is heterozygote for the gene. Let's take an example.

If our mother has blue eyes she has two genes for blue eyes. Blue eyes are recessive so she must be homozygote for the gene for blue eyes which we will label b-b. Our father has brown eyes. Brown eyes are dominant, which means that since brown eyes are dominant only one of his two genes has to be for brown eyes. He could either be a heterozygote, B-b, where B is the dominant allele and b is the recessive allele for brown eyes, or a homozygote, B-B. We can't tell the difference. The phenotype, "brown eyes," is the same.

Let us assume that our father was heterozygote for brown eyes, meaning that he had one gene for brown eyes and one for blue eyes. Then, if mom and dad had four children, on average, since one gene for eye color must come from mom and one from dad, two children would have blue eyes and two children would have brown eyes. Our mother would always give us a gene for blue eyes, but there was a fifty-fifty chance that we would get the gene for blue eyes from dad. On the other hand if both of our father's gene were for brown eyes, in other words he was homozygote for B, all four children would have brown eyes.

Alpha 1 antitrypsin deficiency is the most common genetic cause of emphysema. It is due to a mutation on the autosomal SERPINA 1 gene found on chromosome 14. The SERPINA 1 gene is *codominant* which means that having just one gene will cause at least mild disease. Both bad genes are needed to get severe disease. There are three possible alleles on the SERPINA 1 gene. The first is M which is the normal allele. The second is S which causes mild disease. The third is Z which causes severe disease. A person who has two Z alleles has an extremely high risk of getting emphysema and dying young because of it while a person with MZ or SZ will likely have mild disease, or in many cases, no disease at all.

The condition was first described in 1963. There are approximately 3.4 million people with alpha 1 antitrypsin deficiency worldwide. But the condition is underreported. Very few doctors do genetic testing on every patient with any form of COPD. Alpha 1 antitrypsin deficiency can even cause asthma! Thus, it is now recommended that all patients with COPD including those with **poorly controlled** asthma be tested for alpha 1 antitrypsin deficiency.

While the disease affects mainly the lungs in adults and the liver in children it can also even affect the blood vessels causing a vasculitis as well as fat cells causing a panniculitis, or inflammation of fatty tissue. Alpha 1 antitrypsin is synthesized in the liver and then enters the blood to travel to the lung and other organs. If it is deficient in the liver, toxic proteins accumulate around the liver cells, killing them and forming plaques which lead ultimately to cirrhosis. If you are a child and have the ZZ gene, you have about a 25% chance of developing cirrhosis during your childhood.

In an adult, alpha 1 antitrypsin deficiency causes panlobular emphysema. How does that come about? With inflammation of the lung, whether it be caused by a simple case of bronchitis or by smoking, the neutrophils and macrophages produce trypsin, an enzyme which breaks down protein debris whether it is the protein of bacteria, viruses, or dead cells. Once the inflammation is controlled there are, in normal people, antitrypsins which turn off the trypsin. If there are no antitrypsins then the trypsin attacks the normal lung tissue, destroying it. Emphysema is the result.

Other factors affect whether the patient will get COPD. Smoking is easily the most important. If the patient is homozygote for the Z allele (ZZ) and is a smoker he or she has a 90% chance of getting COPD while if he or she is a nonsmoker there is only a 65% chance of COPD. *In fact, 30% of patients who are ZZ and don't smoke are healthy.*

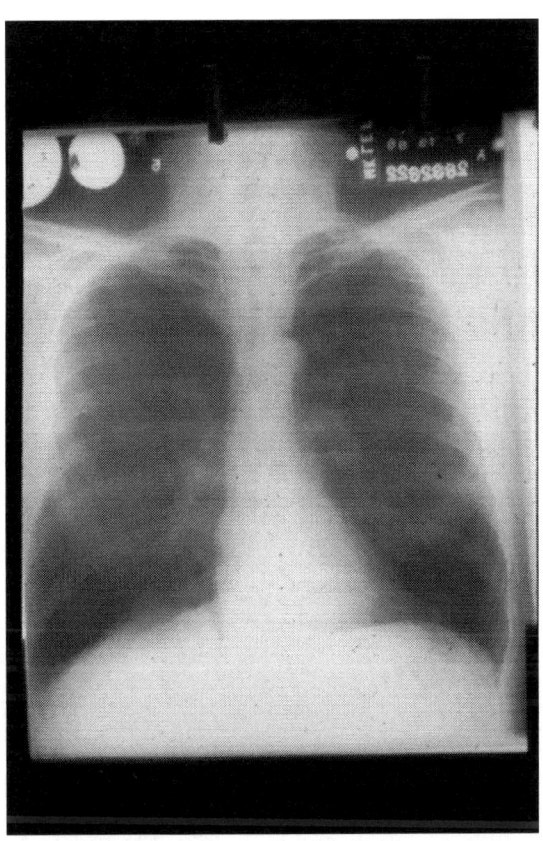

This is a chest x-ray of a patient with alpha 1 antitrypsin deficiency. There is marked flattening of the diaphragms as well as very prominent hila suggesting the presence of cor pulmonale. Most importantly, the emphysema clearly involves mainly the lower lobes. There are no lung markings in the lower lobes at all.

The difference between typical emphysema and emphysema due to alpha 1 antitrypsin deficiency is that the latter condition involves mainly the lower lobes. The lower lobes are where most of our inhaled air, bacteria, tobacco smoke, and other environmental demons go. The lower lobes are also where most of our blood flow goes.

Treatment is available for the condition. It involves giving the patient exogenous alpha 1 antitrypsin intravenously twice a month. It won't cure the disease but it will slow its progression. Because there is an effective treatment, all patients with any form of COPD (except well-controlled asthmatics) should be screened for the disease.

One of the newer recommendations is that Respiratory Therapists will be responsible for ordering blood tests for alpha 1 antitrypsin deficiency when they perform pulmonary function testing which shows that a patient has obstructive lung disease.

Chronic Bronchitis

Unlike emphysema which requires a pathological diagnosis, the diagnosis of chronic bronchitis is clinical. Simply put, it is the presence of a cough for three months of the year for two years in a row. It is most often caused by smoking but certain occupations may be important causes of the disease. Exposure to coal dust and cotton dust increase the risk of chronic bronchitis. The disorder is also common in welders, chemical workers, pottery workers, metal workers, textile workers and in people who work in flour mills. Even air pollution increases the risk of chronic bronchitis.

The patient with typical chronic bronchitis is heavy set, laid back, and blue. He has a low oxygen level, a high level of carbon dioxide, and a high hematocrit. He is part of the "50-50-50 Club". His chest x-ray is usually normal.

Chronic bronchitis is due to inflammation of the bronchi and lung parenchyma which cause *narrowing* of the airways and the *loss of supporting lung structure* which then causes mismatching of ventilation and perfusion resulting in hypoxemia which, if unchecked, causes pulmonary hypertension, cor pulmonale, and death.

In fact, cor pulmonale occurs earlier in the course of chronic bronchitis than it does in the patient with emphysema. Unlike the patient with emphysema who has cor pulmonale due to the progressive loss of capillaries and blood vessels, cor pulmonale in the patient with chronic bronchitis is due to hypoxemia. The hypoxia causes vasospasm which causes the cor pulmonale. Correct the hypoxia and the cor pulmonale goes away.

A major difference between emphysema and chronic bronchitis is that emphysema is associated with *increased dead space* whereas chronic bronchitis, because it causes airway narrowing due to mucous and inflammation, is associated with *physiologic shunting*. The increased dead space doesn't affect the blood oxygen level much if at all, but the shunting affects the blood oxygen and carbon dioxide a lot.

The severity of the disease is based on pulmonary function testing. All patients diagnosed with chronic bronchitis must have an FEV1/FVC ratio less than 70%. Mild disease is an FEV1 of 80-100% of predicted; moderate disease is an FEV1 of 50-80%; severe disease is an FEV 1 of 30-50%; very severe disease is an FEV1 of less than 30%.

The treatment for chronic bronchitis is to first assess and monitor the disease and its progression by using chest x-rays, pulmonary function testing, as well as the six-minute walk which is an excellent tool to evaluate the physiologic status of the patient. The patient must also reduce his or her risk factors. Smoking should stop. The patient's work history needs to be examined in detail to determine if he or she is exposed to toxins at work. Lastly, the patient needs to get both the pneumococcal and influenza vaccines. Moreover, the physician must manage both the stable disease and exacerbations of the disease.

The primary goals of management of the stable patient are to prevent progression of the disease, reduce symptoms, increase functional abilities, and prevent exacerbations of the illness

The management of the stable patient always begins getting the patient to stop smoking. Then step therapy is applied following the GOLD Workshop Report. The medications which are used are similar to the agents we use in the asthmatic and include inhaled B adrenergic agents, inhaled anticholinergic agents, theophyllines and inhaled steroids. Oxygen therapy and pulmonary rehabilitation are also very important in treating the patient with chronic bronchitis.

Asthma

Asthma is defined functionally or physiologically as "reversible airways obstructive disease". In other words, there must be a 12% improvement in the FEV1 following the administration of a B adrenergic agent such as albuterol.

Pathologically, asthma is characterized by hypertrophy of the bronchial smooth muscle, thickening of the basement membrane, a marked increase in the number of gland cells and submucosal blood vessels and a pronounced eosinophilic infiltrate in the bronchial wall. The airway is narrowed because of the thickened bronchial wall. It is filled with tiny casts of the airways called Curschmann's spirals. At autopsy the lungs don't collapse when the chest is opened and copious amounts of thick gelatinous mucous oozes from the airways.

There are many, many causes of asthma. Asthma is at least in part a genetic disease. It is clearly related to a family history of allergy or atopy. And we have already noted that alpha 1 antitrypsin deficiency can present as asthma. But it is also related to tobacco abuse and certain infections, including the Respiratory Syncytial Virus in children and a Mycoplasma infection in young adults. Obesity and reflux esophagitis can cause treatable forms of asthma. Lastly certain chemicals including Aspirin, Tartrazines, and Metasulfites can cause asthma.

Asthma can be divided into two groups: allergic or extrinsic asthma and non-allergic or intrinsic asthma.

Extrinsic asthma usually affects children and teenagers. It is characterized by a high eosinophil count and increased IgE in the blood. It is associated with atopy or the tendency towards allergies. Atopic people often have allergic rhinitis and eczema. The allergen combines with IgE molecules which are bound to the mast cells in the lung. The mast cells then release histamines and leukotrienes which cause the intense inflammatory reaction as well as the smooth muscle contraction.

Intrinsic asthma affects adults. The IgE and eosinophil count are normal. It is not associated with atopy.

But what do we mean by atopy and hypersensitivity? It is an immune response that is "over the top". It is an immune response out of proportion to the exposure to the allergen.

There are four types of **hypersensitivity**. Type 1, which is the type seen in hay fever and extrinsic asthma, is mediated by IgE and is called **"immediate hypersensitivity"**. Th2 lymphocytes, in response to a large allergen load, secrete large amounts of specific IgE which then binds to receptors on the mast cells and basophils. When the large number of IgE molecules on the mast cells bind to the allergen, they deform the mast cell which releases chemicals including histamines and arachidonic acid found in the cellular granules. These chemicals cause bronchospasm, vasodilation as well as the production of leukotrienes. The activated Th2 lymphocytes and activated mast cells also secrete IL-5 (interleukin 5) which results in the increased production and activation of eosinophils. IL-4 and IL-13 are also involved. The eosinophils then cause a **delayed allergic reaction** hours later. Twenty percent of the world's population suffer from atopy or "immediate hypersensitivity". Why? Likely in order to prevent worm infestation. Th2 mediated asthma is the most common form of asthma.

Type 2 hypersensitivity involves the antibody directly attacking normal tissue resulting in inflammation. Myasthenia gravis, a neurological disease, is an example of this. Type 3 hypersensitivity involves the formation of an antigen-antibody complex in the blood. These complexes are called "immune complexes." Whenever we have an infection we form some of these complexes but the body is able to clear them. However, if the number of complexes is large, it may overwhelm the defenses and the complexes may be deposited in tissues such as the kidneys or the joints or the small blood vessels. Systemic Lupus Erythematosus is an example of this type. This disease is characterized by renal failure, arthritis, disease of the heart valves and brain.

Lastly, Type 4 hypersensitivity is a **cellular immunity** mediated by T-lymphocytes, especially CD4 lymphocytes. This type of hypersensitivity is associated with psoriasis, rheumatoid arthritis, multiple sclerosis, and even eczema. Characteristically, cellular immunity requires 24 to 48 hours to become manifest (delayed type hypersensitivity). An example of this type is the PPD test used to detect the presence of antibodies to the tuberculosis bacterium.

The symptoms of asthma include cough, shortness of breath, tightness in the chest and wheezing.

There are two types of cough which readily point to a diagnosis of asthma. The first is the exercise-induced cough which occurs a few minutes after STOPPING exercise. When we exercise we produce both adrenaline, which is a bronchodilator, and histamine, which is a bronchoconstrictor. When we stop exercise the adrenaline levels drop but the histamine levels remain elevated and asthma develops. The second type of cough is the night cough which generally occurs in the middle of the night as opposed to the night cough of congestive heart failure which generally occurs an hour or so after the patient lies down.

Physical findings in an acutely ill patient include hyperinflation which is often quite dramatic. The patient may sit in the tripod position and use the accessory muscles of respiration. Breath sounds may be decreased. Wheezing may be present. But in an office setting the patient who is in between attacks of asthma, may have no abnormal physical findings at all.

The chest x-ray is normal in most patients with asthma. The diagnosis is established by the *pulmonary function studies*. If the patient has active disease, his FEV1 should be reduced out of proportion to his FVC. Having the patient inhale a B adrenergic agent should result in at least a 12% increase in the FEV1 or FVC. If the pulmonary function testing is *normal*, the Methacholine Challenge can be done. Methacholine is similar to acetyl choline, the chemical released by the parasympathetic nervous system which causes bronchoconstriction. Methacholine also causes bronchoconstriction. Tiny, graded amounts of methacholine are given by inhalation to the patient and the change in FEV1 is monitored. If the FEV1 drops 20%, the diagnosis of asthma is made. The test is 95% sensitive and 95% specific. No other test comes close. False positives can occur in someone who has allergic rhinitis or in someone who recently had the flu.

Asthma must be treated by addressing both bronchoconstriction as well as inflammation. Bronchodilators are used to treat bronchospasm. These agents include B adrenergic agents, anticholinergic agents and theophyllines. Steroids, leukotriene modifiers and anti-IgE are used to treat the inflammation.

Cyclic AMP (adenosine monophosphate) causes bronchodilation of the airways. It is produced from ATP by the enzyme *adenyl cyclase* and it is broken down into adenosine monophosphate by the enzyme *phosphodiesterase*. The B adrenergic agents increase the activity of adenyl cyclase thus increasing cyclic AMP. On the other hand the theophyllines block the enzyme phosphodiesterase preventing the breakdown of cyclic AMP thus increasing its level.

The enzyme *guanylate cyclase* increases the level of cyclic-GMP which causes bronchoconstriction. The anticholinergic agents block the enzyme and thus decrease the cyclic-GMP (cyclic guanosine monophosphate) causing bronchodilation.

Since B adrenergic agents, theophyllines, and anticholinergics all act on different enzymes, they can be used together to treat asthma.

Steroids, such as prednisone and inhaled cortisones, increase the sensitivity of the lung to the B adrenergic agents. In addition they have direct anti-inflammatory properties. The leukotriene modifiers also block the inflammatory process but are far less effective than steroids. Steroids taken by mouth, however, have very serious side effects including osteoporosis, cataracts, obesity, and infections.

Anti-IgE agents are chemicals which bind directly to IgE on the mast cells so that the allergen can't attach to the cell preventing the release of the histamines and leukotrienes.

There are several new specific anti-leukotriene agents. They are all antibodies and bind to the specific leukotriene (IL-5, IL4 or IL-13) blocking its action. These agents are generally given intravenously but are proving quite effective in resistant asthma. They can decrease the risk of asthmatic exacerbations by up to 50%.

Aspirin causes a particularly severe form of asthma in susceptible individuals. Even tiny amounts of aspirin can set off an asthmatic attack which does not respond to B adrenergic agents, anticholinergic agents or even steroids. Aspirin-exacerbated respiratory disease affects 7% of asthmatics and 15% of severe asthmatics. The hallmarks are sinusitis, nasal polyps and asthma. Other symptoms include the total loss of smell as well as asthma precipitated by red wine or beer. The median-age of onset is 30 years. It is never seen in the newborn or in Chinese though it does not appear to be a genetic disorder. Nevertheless 2/3rds of patients are atopic or allergic. Only drugs which can access the small COX-1 channel such as Aspirin, Naprosyn and Ibuprofen can cause the disorder. COX-2 inhibitors (Mobic and Celebrex) can't cause the disorder. The treatment is "aspirin desensitization". Basically, the patient takes 325 mg of ASA daily. The first day precipitates a severe reaction; from then on the patient does well. However the patient can't miss more than one day.

Yellow dye no. 5, which is used as a food coloring agent, and Metasulfites, which are used as preservatives in beer, wine, and salad bars, can even cause asthma.

Allergic aspergillosis is uncommon but not rare. It is due to the fungus aspergillosis which colonizes the bronchial lining and provokes an allergic response. The patient develops asthma but also has changes of bronchiectasis with thickened airways and "tram lines" and even a pneumonic infiltrate on the chest x-ray. The hallmark of the disease is the presence of sputum "so thick you can chew it." The diagnosis is established by culturing the organism in the sputum or by finding antibodies to the organism in the blood. The only treatment that works is steroids which must be given for life. Antifungal agents may be needed as well.

Bronchiectasis

Bronchiectasis is an uncommon disease. It has many known causes including cystic fibrosis as well as immune-deficiency states such as AIDS.

Like chronic bronchitis it is defined clinically. The patient has a chronic cough productive of copious amounts (more than 20 cc a day) of purulent phlegm. Pathologically there is permanent severe dilation and distortion of bronchi and bronchioles.

The etiology is extensive. Certainly genetic diseases top the list and include Cystic fibrosis, Congenital Immunodeficiency Syndrome, Dyskinetic Cilia Syndrome and Kartagener's Syndrome. Infectious diseases, especially Mycobacterium avium infection, can also cause the disease. HIV is becoming a more common cause as well. Autoimmune diseases such as Rheumatoid Arthritis, Lupus erythematosis, and Sjogren's disease are less frequent causes.

The most common cause of bronchiectasis in children and young adults is Cystic Fibrosis. It is the most common inherited disease in America. It affects Whites three times as often as Hispanics, five times more often than Blacks and ten times more often than Asians. About one in every two hundred Whites is a carrier of the mutation. It is an autosomal recessive genetic disorder involving a site on the 7th chromosome. This means that you must have both genes for cystic fibrosis in order to get the disease. Unlike alpha 1 antitrypsin deficiency, cystic fibrosis can be caused by many different alleles. There are hundreds of abnormal alleles that have been identified. The most common is phe508del. The gene involved controls the chloride ion channel regulator. When the chloride channel is blocked the movement of water in and out of the cell is impaired. The skin tastes salty and the airway mucous, the pancreatic secretions, and the mucous in the gut become thick. These changes cause bronchiectasis in the lungs, pancreatic failure and meconium ileus in babies.

The disease can present shortly after birth with a meconium ileus. The stool is hard and thick and the baby is unable to pass it. He or she develops severe abdominal pain and vomiting. If the child does not develop a meconium ileus, then the disease will present as asthma or recurrent bronchitis while the child is still quite young. The diagnosis is made with the sweat test, which is still the gold standard test, or with genetic testing.

Symptoms of the disease include a persistent cough which is productive of more than 20 ccs of purulent sputum a day, hemoptysis and shortness of breath, as well as symptoms related to chronic sinusitis and cor pulmonale. Physical findings include nasal polyps, fetid breath, coarse crackles, clubbing and signs of cor pulmonale in the advanced case.

The chest x-ray is often diagnostic. The lungs are hyperinflated but, in addition, there are areas of pulmonary fibrosis or scarring, along with infiltrates suggestive of pneumonia or atelectasis. There may be "tram lines" which are thickened bronchial walls and cystic lesions often partially fluid filled.

The diagnosis is established with a high resolution CAT scan of the chest. It is 90% sensitive and 90% specific. Typical findings include cystic airways with tram lines, cysts with air fluid levels called "signet rings" and mucoid impactions.

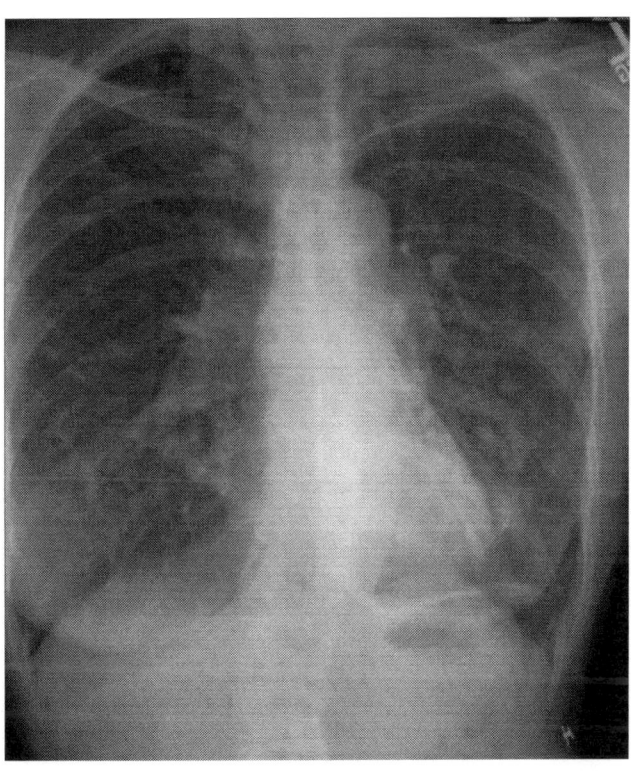

Typical chest x-ray of a patient with bronchiectasis. There is flattening of the diaphragms as well as widened rib spacing consistent with hyperinflation. In addition there is a "dirty" appearing lung parenchyma due to fibrosis. There is also an infiltrate along the left heart border. The hila are large due to cor pulmonale.

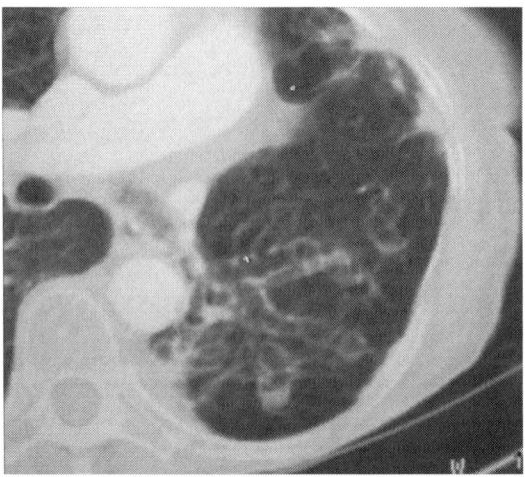

The CAT scan shows large dilated bronchi involving the left lower lobe. This is so-called "cylindrical bronchiectasis".

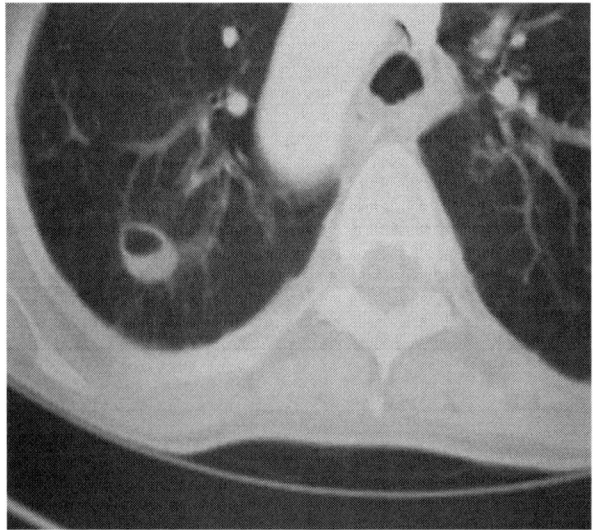

A "signet ring sign" is seen in the right lower lobe of this patient.

The patient's pulmonary function studies show a mixed restrictive and obstructive pattern.

Evaluation of the patient with suspected bronchiectasis includes performing the sweat test even in the adult patient, testing for HIV, and obtaining an Immunoglobulin panel, IgE level, sputum and serology for aspergillosis and a sputum for AFB.

Treatment for bronchiectasis is at best problematic. There are no cures. The most important part of the treatment plan is intense attention to pulmonary toilet including postural drainage and percussion. B adrenergic agents and monthly antibiotics, especially azithromycin may be helpful. Dornase, an inhaled agent which breaks down DNA molecules is approved for patients with Cystic Fibrosis. Nebulized antibiotics, specifically tobramycin, are also being used with some success. If the patient has localized disease surgery may be helpful as well. Lastly, lung transplantation is an option for the younger patient.

Newer therapies are available for **Cystic Fibrosis**. The mainstay of treatment remains good pulmonary toilet including postural drainage and percussion as well as the use of inhaled hypertonic saline and inhaled Dornase or Pulmozyme, an enzyme which breaks down the DNA in the airway debris reducing the viscosity of the mucous, making it easier to expel. The newest therapies, all developed in the last ten years are the CFTR correctors which move CFTR protein to the correct place on the surface of cells. Once there, they work by opening the CFTR channel, facilitating the transport of chloride and sodium (salt) in and out of cells. There are three different types of "correctors". All are given orally and when used together improve the FEV1 and sweat chloride in 90% of patients (those with the allele Phe508del which makes up 90% of patients with CF).[4]

1. Tezacaftor binds the CFTR protein increasing the amount of mature CFTR available at the cell surface
2. Ivacaftor increases the channel-gating activity of the CFTR protein
3. Both VX-659 and VX 445 have an additive effect on the other agents

If all else fails then a lung transplant can give several years of productive life to the patient.

Recently, several studies have pointed to the importance of the lung's microbiome and the mucociliary ladder in the pathogenesis of bronchiectasis and exacerbations of COPD. Normally, we all aspirate tiny amounts of oral secretions filled with bacteria, especially anaerobes. We also eliminate some of the bacteria. There is thus a "steady state" relationship between aspiration and elimination. The mucous lining are major airways is thin which allows us to be able to readily clear secretions. If the mucous becomes thick because of dehydration, usually due to infection, it will pool in puddles along the airway. If the puddles are in the large airways we can cough them up. But if the puddles are in the small airways they become the nidus for infection. The oral anaerobic bacteria (bacteria that don't require oxygen to live) thrive in the puddles. These organisms release chemicals which allow other aerobic bacteria such as pseudomonas and staphylococcus to grow. Treatment must be directed at hydrating the mucous layer. Inhaled hypertonic saline is, at present, the most effective therapy. Acetyl cysteine has NOT been shown to be effective at all.

---

[4] J. C. Davies, et. al., and D. Keating, et. al., both articles in the NEJM, volume 379, number 17 for the week of October 25, 2018, pages 1599 to 1620.

IMPORTANT CONCEPTS TO REMEMBER FROM THIS LECTURE

1. Asthma is defined as:

    Reversible airways obstructive disease

2. The diffusion (DCO) is normal in obstructive lung diseases except in patients with:

    Emphysema

3. In the typical patient with emphysema the blood gases are:

    Normal

4. A patient with severe chronic bronchitis is characterized by being part of the "50-50-50 Club". What does that mean?

    The pO2 is 50; the pCO2 is 50; the hematocrit is 50.

5. Bronchiectasis is characterized by:

    The production of more than 20 cc of purulent phlegm daily

Lecture Seventeen

Restrictive Lung Diseases

When we think about restrictive lung disease we focus our minds on disorders such as pulmonary fibrosis, sarcoidosis, asbestosis, and many other conditions in which the normal lung parenchyma is replaced with scar tissue. But restrictive disease needs to be more inclusive. Even a stroke, a disease in which part of the brain is destroyed, will cause a 15% decrease in vital capacity.

We need to be aware of all the conditions that can cause the loss of lung volume:

Neuromuscular Diseases
    Central nervous system
    Upper motor neuron diseases
    Lower motor neuron diseases
    Diseases of the neuro-muscular junction
    Diseases of muscle
Chest Wall Disorders
    Obesity
    Kyphoscoliosis
Diseases of the pleura
    Pneumothorax, pleural effusion
Diseases of the lung
    Acute including pneumonia and pulmonary edema
    Chronic interstitial lung diseases
        Idiopathic pulmonary fibrosis
        Sarcoidosis
        Hypersensitivity pneumonia
        Occupational diseases
            Asbestosis
            Silicosis
            Coal Worker's Disease

Even this table is incomplete. In fact, there are at least two hundred causes of restrictive disease. But our table provides us with an outline for this lecture.

Neuromuscular Diseases in General

We need to know a little bit about the anatomy of the nervous system. When we decide to kick a ball, the appropriate upper motor neurons in the outer layer of the brain called the grey matter fire, sending a signal down the axon of the nerve, crossing left to right and right to left in the medulla then heading down the anterior and lateral tracts of the spinal cord till they reach the appropriate level where the fibers connect with lower motor neurons in the anterior horn of the spinal cord. These lower motor neurons then join together outside the spinal cord forming a peripheral nerve. Finally the lower motor neuron communicates with the appropriate muscle at the neuromuscular junction. The nerve releases acetyl choline which travels across the junction and binds to a receptor on the muscle. This causes the muscle to release calcium into the sarcoplasmic reticulum which then excites the actin and myosin fibrils causing them to contract and we kick the ball.

The motor and large sensory neurons are covered in a myelin sheath. The sheath does two things. It provides nourishment for the axons. But even more importantly the myelin sheath speeds transmission of the electrical signal from the brain to the muscle. Instead of the signal travelling micron by micron down the nerve, the signal hops its way down the nerve from one Node of Ranvier, which is an area of the nerve not covered with myelin, to the next Node of Ranvier.

Not all nerves are covered with myelin. The nerves that convey our position in space, the nerves that tell us whether something is hot or cold, the nerves of smell and taste, and many others have no myelin. Conduction is much slower. If you put your hand on a hot skillet you will hurt from the pain before the signal for hot gets to your brain.

Lastly, we need to understand a little bit about reflexes. Reflexes do not need the brain. When the doctor strikes the tendon just below the kneecap, a sensory nerve signal is sent from the tendon to the spinal cord which interacts directly with a motor neuron in the spinal cord which then sends a signal to the muscle which contracts. No brain required. No thinking required. The reflex involves only the lower motor neurons. But upper motor neurons from the cerebral cortex can inhibit or turn off the reflex. When the doctor hits the tendon below the knee, the brain can say, "I am not going to have a reflex," and the reflex won't happen. If the upper motor neurons are not functional, the reflex will be markedly enhanced. The doctor had better get out of the way.

Central Nervous System Lesions

Certainly, the most common lesion of the central nervous system is a stroke. The motor cortex is supplied by the middle cerebral artery. If the artery is plugged by a clot or if the artery ruptures due to an aneurysm, the motor cortex will die and one side of the body will be paralyzed.

Most strokes are due to atrial fibrillation. Atrial fibrillation means that the atria are contracting like a bag of worms. Blood pools in the dilated left atrium and over time forms a clot. Then, suddenly, the clot is let loose, passes through the left ventricle on its way to the brain where it lodges, most often, in the middle cerebral artery. This is called an ischemic stroke. The brain is deprived of blood and appears white. The stroke can also be due to the rupture of a Berry Aneurysm, which is a dilated artery in the brain. When it ruptures or leaks, blood pours out into the delicate brain tissue, killing the nearby tissue. This is called a hemorrhagic stroke. Importantly, Berry Aneurysms are hereditary. If your grandpa died of a hemorrhagic stroke, best let your doctor know!

Either way, clinically, the patient's face is paralyzed on the same side as the lesion but his or her body is paralyzed on the opposite side. In other words, a stroke affecting the right side of the brain will cause right facial weakness but left sided paralysis of the arm and leg.

The treatment of an ischemic stroke is to unclog the artery as soon as possible, within six hours if you can but certainly within fifteen hours. The treatment of a hemorrhagic stroke is prevention. Find the Berry Aneurysm and eliminate it before the stroke happens.

Most studies have shown that strokes reduce the vital capacity, FEV1, and peak expiratory flow by about 15% but a recent study showed that patients with a right-sided weakness are much more affected than patients with left-sided weakness. The decrease in pulmonary function is related to the decreased muscle activity on the affected side.

Multiple Sclerosis (MS) is an autoimmune disease which affects mainly young women. It is twice as common in women as it is in men. It can begin at any age. The further you live from the equator the more likely you are to get the disease. It affects about 8 people per 100,000 in the US but 80 people per 100,000 in Europe and 1600 people per 100,000 in certain northern European countries. Smoking also increases the risk as does having a family history of multiple sclerosis although the disease does not appear to be inherited.

MS is caused by the destruction of the myelin protective sheathing resulting in the formation of plaques. The disease can affect any part of the central nervous system and any myelinated nerve fiber. Thus, the symptoms and pulmonary function findings are protean. Usually the disease begins in the eye with a temporary episode of blindness and then comes and goes over many years, first here, then there. Each time the patient becomes a little more impaired. The disease can wax and wane twenty or more years, in fact, before the patient dies. Sensation as well as motor function is involved. There usually is often cognitive impairment as well.

The treatment is cortisone for acute flares of the disease. In addition plasmapheresis has been used successfully. Finally, disease modifying agents similar to what has been used in rheumatoid arthritis have been shown recently to prevent or at least slow the progression of the disease.

Primarily Upper Motor Neuron Disease

The most common disease in this group is **Amyotrophic Lateral Sclerosis** (ALS). If you are older than I am it is "Lou Gehrig's Disease." If you are younger than I it is "Stephen Hawking's Disease." Either way it is a progressive neurologic disease involving at first the upper motor neurons. Most of the patients with ALS are men in their 60's or 70's. About 10% have a family history of the disease.

The illness begins with muscle weakness which can affect any part of the body. The disease slowly progresses with more and more muscles affected. Finally the brainstem is affected. Speech and swallowing become impaired. Patients generally die of pneumonia due to aspiration after just a few years.

Sensation is NOT affected but there may be mild cognitive impairment in up to a third of the patients. The main physical signs are hyperreflexia, fasciculations (the muscle looks like a bag of worms rolling about), and muscle wasting. When the upper motor neuron dies, the patient develops increased reflexes and fasciculations. The lower motor nerves are involved as well. When they die the muscles they innervate die. The disease is diagnosed when there are both signs of upper and lower motor disease without any other explanation

Pulmonary function studies show restrictive lung disease. The total lung capacity, vital capacity and FEV1 are reduced but the residual volume is increased because the patient can't get the air out due to muscle weakness. Diffusion is normal.

There is no cure for the disease but recently a new medication, Riluzole, has been shown to slow disease progression by about 2-3 months.

Respiratory therapists play an important role in treating the disease. Many patients with ALS will elect to use non-invasive ventilation and even full ventilator support. In addition, postural drainage and suctioning are especially important in the care of the patient with ALS.

Primarily Lower Motor Neuron Disease

There are two diseases that affect the lower motor neuron. The most common disorder in this category is **Guillain-Barre** (GB) which affects all the myelinated nerves. Unlike Multiple Sclerosis the disease is nearly completely reversible over time. It is often called "Ascending Paralysis" because it starts in the legs and works its way up to finally involve the brain stem.

It affects both the motor and sensory nerves but does not interfere with cognition.

The disease can occur at any age in both men and women equally, but is more severe when it occurs in the older adult. It is an autoimmune disease, which simply put means that the body's own immune system is attacking its own nerves. It often begins after a Campylobacter infection which is a bacterial infection that causes gastroenteritis. It can also occur after a flu shot. A few weeks after the infection or vaccination, the patient develops numbness or tingling in the feet followed by progressive weakness, first in the legs, then in the arms, until finally the patient becomes paralyzed. The disease peaks at about 2 to 3 weeks and then improves. Generally there is at least 90% recovery.

The diagnosis is made by getting the typical history and, if necessary, doing a lumbar puncture and obtaining cerebrospinal fluid which will show normal cells but increased protein.

The treatment is either plasmapheresis in which the abnormal antibodies are removed in a process similar to dialysis or giving intravenous gamma globulin (IV-IG), which binds to the abnormal antigen causing the disease, preventing it from binding to the patient's own antibodies (competitive inhibition). Both therapies are equally effective.

About a third of patients will require ventilator support for a week or two.

The second lower motor neuron disease is **poliomyelitis**. Prior to 1950, Polio was the most common neuromuscular condition resulting in respiratory failure. In the developed world cases are rare today and are usually due to the vaccine itself (About 1 case per 2.5 million doses). There have been no cases in the United States since 1999. Polio is due to a single stranded RNA virus which attacks the anterior horn of the spinal cord killing the lower motor neurons and causing a flaccid paralysis. The illness begins as a mild pharyngitis associated with malaise and fever, followed by muscle weakness. The cerebrospinal fluid shows increased protein and white cells. Paralysis is unusual but of those who develop neurologic symptoms 25% will require ventilator assistance during the acute illness. Before the Salk vaccine was developed one whole floor of the largest hospital in the world, St. Mary's Hospital in Rochester Minnesota, was a sea of Iron Lungs.

About 25% of patients who have a history of polio in the past develop new neurological symptoms, such as weakness, 25-40 years after the acute illness. These new symptoms include muscular weakness due to degeneration of re-innervated motor units. The disease is characterized by weakness, fatigue, muscle fasciculation, and pain associated with muscle atrophy. Generally the illness plateaus after 1 to 10 years.

While polio was devastating to millions and millions of people, it did usher in the use of ventilators. Of course, we all have seen photos of the Iron Lung, an external ventilator. But in addition, the Erickson ventilator was introduced as well. This ventilator was basically a piston with a fixed volume that delivered air to the patient through a cuffless endotracheal tube. The patient exhaled around the tube. It was of course the earliest form synchronized intermittent mechanical ventilation or SIMV. The Erickson ventilator had the added advantage of being able to slide under the patient's bed.

Recently a new theory has been proposed to explain the cause of these degenerative neurological diseases such as polio, Guillain-Barre, ALS, and MS. All of these diseases were very uncommon prior to the 1950's. A few scientists have suggested that it was the attention to hygiene at the turn of the 20th century that caused the outbreak of the diseases. Certainly polio is caused by a virus and Guillain-Barre is definitely related to the bacterium Campylobacter. These scientists have suggested that before the 20th century babies were exposed to common pathogens while their immune system was being developed. They developed normal antibodies to fight the diseases. If however, they were not exposed early on, when they finally came in contact with these infectious agents, they developed faulty antibodies which attacked not only the invader but also the normal neurologic tissues. The scientists are not suggesting that we should send our infants into the swamp before they are six months old. Rather they are suggesting we need to find vaccines to prevent these diseases. When I was a child, I did not mind playing in the swamp, though of course, my mother did object strenuously.

Disease of the Neuromuscular Junction (NMJ).

Myasthenia gravis is the most common disorder of the NMJ. It is also an autoimmune disorder. The neuromuscular junction is complex. The nerve innervating the muscle releases acetyl choline which travels to receptors on the muscle cells and binds to them, deforming the surface of the cell. The change in the surface configuration results in the release of Calcium which travels to the sarcoplasmic reticulum where it initiates the contraction of the actin and myosin fibrils. After binding to the receptor, the acetyl choline is destroyed quickly by the enzyme cholinesterase. The muscle relaxes and the whole process can now be repeated.

Patients with Myasthenia gravis have fewer and deformed receptors. The first batch of acetyl choline binds to the receptors but there are no receptors left for additional binding. Thus, even though the nerve is pouring out acetyl choline in order to make the muscle contract, it just won't happen. The muscles become less and less responsive till finally they don't work at all.

Typically the patient presents first with double vision (diplopia) or with droopy eyelids (ptosis). The muscle weakness then spreads downward to larger and larger muscle groups. Rest relieves the symptoms for a brief period.

The diagnosis is made finding typical antibodies against the acetyl choline receptor in the patient's serum. If the patient has ptosis, the "ice test" can be done. Putting ice on the eye with ptosis will at least temporarily correct the ptosis. Lastly, the Tensilon test can be done. Tensilon is a cholinesterase inhibitor. By blocking the cholinesterase the level of acetyl choline is increased. This overwhelms the receptor system and the patient's muscles will be stronger, at least temporarily. Tensilon can cause asthma and other side effects and is rarely done today.

The disease is treated with cholinesterase inhibitors. During an acute flare of the disease, steroids are used as well. The disease is often associated with tumors of the thymus gland and, sometimes, removing the thymus gland (thymectomy) can be helpful.

Diseases of Muscle

The most common muscle disorder is **polymyositis** or **dermatomyositis**. It is an autoimmune disease closely related to Systemic Lupus Erythematosis (SLE) and Rheumatoid Arthritis (RA). It involves the proximal muscles of the arms and legs which become inflamed and tender. The patient develops generalized fatigue. Sometimes even swallowing is affected. Like SLE, it is more common in women than in men and generally affects younger people. If there a skin rash, generally seen over the knuckles, associated with the polymyositis, the patient has dermatomyositis.

The diagnosis is made with a muscle biopsy and the treatment is cortisone.

Chest Wall Disorders

Morbid obesity, that is a BMI (body mass index) greater than 45, is associated with restrictive lung disease. But interestingly not all morbidly obese patients will have abnormal lung function. Why some patients do and some don't is ill understood. Classically there is decreased total lung capacity, residual volume, and vital capacity. The functional residual capacity is decreased because of the stiff chest wall. **Diffusing capacity is however increased** in most but not all morbidly obese patients. The increased diffusion is believed to be due to increased blood volume seen in the obese patient which likely improves the relationship between ventilation and perfusion in the lung. Some studies have shown, however, decreased diffusion in a few patients. In addition, morbidly obese patients with hypoxemia likely have increased mismatching of ventilation and perfusion.

Kyphoscoliosis is characterized by both a forward bend and a lateral bend of the thoracic spine. This puts the intercostal muscles, the abdominal muscles, and even the diaphragm at a disadvantage. In addition with time, osteoarthritis develops and the chest wall becomes rigid. The combination of muscle weakness and a rigid chest wall results in restrictive lung disease with a decrease in total lung capacity, normal or increased residual volume and decreased functional residual capacity. Diffusion is normal.

Interstitial Lung Diseases (ILD)

There are more than 170 types of interstitial lung disease. For most patients, the main symptom is shortness of breath although in Usual Interstitial Pneumonitis (UIP or UIP-F), there is also a severe, unremitting, irritating dry cough. In almost all patients with ILD, the breath sounds are decreased and there are fine inspiratory crackles which are called "Velcro Rales" because they sound like two pieces of Velcro being pulled apart. Some patients, especially those with Usual Interstitial Pneumonitis or Asbestosis, may have clubbing. The pulmonary function tests are fairly uniform and show, because of the stiff lungs, decreased total lung capacity, decreased functional residual capacity, decreased residual volume and decreased diffusion. The Chest x-ray is often helpful in establishing the diagnosis. Sarcoidosis and Hypersensitivity Pneumonitis are generally disease of the upper lung field diseases whereas Usual Interstitial Pneumonitis and Asbestosis are lower lung field diseases. In most cases the diagnosis is made by biopsy except in Usual Interstitial Pneumonitis-Fibrosis where the diagnosis can be made with the high resolution CAT scan of the chest and a biopsy is no longer needed in most cases.

The most common types of interstitial lung disease are: Usual Interstitial Pneumonitis-fibrosis (UIP), Nonspecific Interstitial Pneumonitis (NSIP), Hypersensitivity Pneumonitis (HP), Sarcoidosis and pneumoconiosis such as Asbestosis and Silicosis.

The most common of the interstitial pneumonitides is **Usual Interstitial Pneumonitis-Fibrosis**, a disease of unknown etiology, which results in progressive pulmonary fibrosis. The disease was first described by Hamman and Rich in the late 1930's. The disease involves older individuals, more often male. The older you get the more likely you are to get the disease. The life expectancy after diagnosis is about 2 to 4 years. The most common presenting symptoms are breathlessness and a dry cough. The cough is severe and unremitting. It may bother the patient even more than the shortness of breath. The physical exam shows bibasilar crackles ("Velcro Rales") as well as clubbing late in the course of the disease. Clubbing is seen in 50% and arthritis in about 20% of the patients with UIP. Cyanosis and cor pulmonale occur late. The diagnosis can usually be made by HRCT, which demonstrates: reticular (linear) opacities, traction bronchiectasis, and honeycombing in the lung bases peripherally. Open lung biopsy can confirm the diagnosis if needed: there is obliteration of the lung architecture with prominent smooth muscle bundles admixed with fibrosis and honey combing. The severe lung disease is admixed with areas of normal lung. There is no cure for the disease. Steroids and other drugs used in the past are not only ineffective, they may, in fact, worsen the disease. Recently two new medications, Pirfenidone and Nintedanib, have been introduced which improve the pulmonary function studies but don't appear to affect the patient's life span and don't affect the horrid cough. The only approved treatment at the moment are the new agents, Pirfenidone and Nintedanib, both of which downregulate fibroblast growth factor.

Usual Interstitial Pneumonitis is associated with pulmonary hypertension which may be caused by the disease process itself or may be a separate disease. The most dreaded event in the course of the disease is an Acute Exacerbation. These episodes may occur at any time during the course of the illness and are characterized by a worsening shortness of breath and the presence of new infiltrates on the High Resolution CAT scan. If the new infiltrates are peripheral reticular changes, they may be responsive to steroids. If they are ground glass and multiple, they will not be responsive. The hallmark of an exacerbation is a fall in oxygen level without evidence of an infection despite the presence of leukocytosis on the complete blood count.

UIP has a stepwise course. It is stable for a while; then there is an exacerbation. Then it is stable again followed by another exacerbation. Finally the patient succumbs to the disease. The most common causes of death are respiratory failure in about half the patients, cardiovascular disease in a quarter of the patients, and pneumonia, pulmonary embolism, and lung cancer in the remainder of the patients.

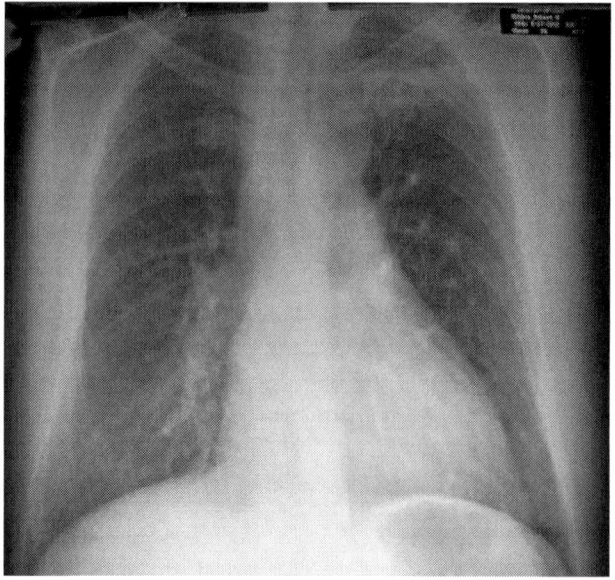

The chest x-ray of a patient with idiopathic or usual interstitial pneumonitis fibrosis showing bibasilar, reticular (meaning linear) densities.

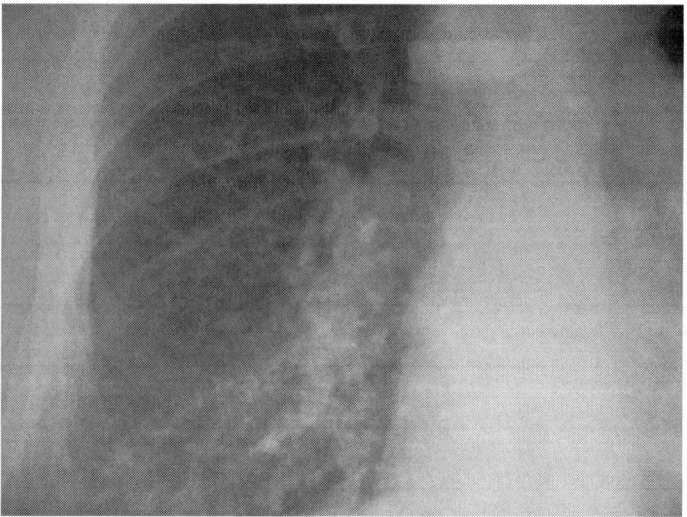

A closer view shows the reticular (linear) markings in detail.

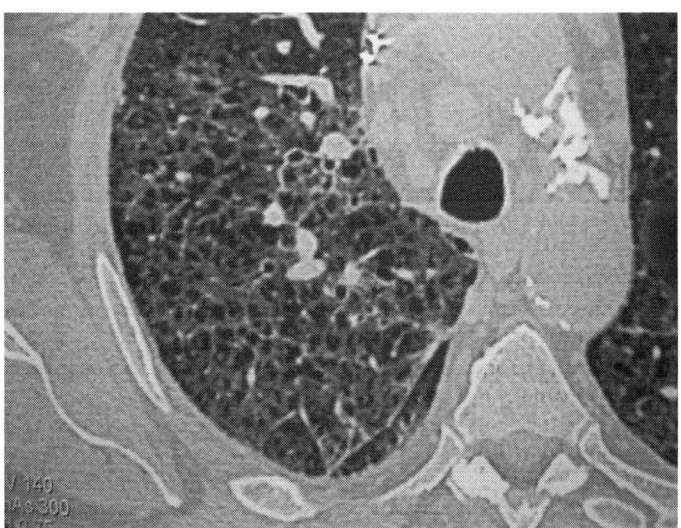

The high resolution CAT scan of a patient with UIP shows the honeycombing and distortion of the bronchial tubes. There is NO ground glass infiltrate. The lesion is also more peripheral in location though in this case the whole lung is involved.

Non-specific interstitial pneumonitis-fibrosis is the second most common type of ILD. It affects both men and women in their late forties and early fifties. There is a more rapid onset of symptoms compared to UIP. Thirty percent will have fever! Clubbing is rarely found. The high resolution CAT scan of the chest is similar to UIP but there is NO honeycombing. Instead there is a ground glass appearance. The biopsy shows a uniform, diffuse interstitial fibrosis with a lymphocytic infiltrate. More than half the patients have associated collagen vascular disorders such as Systemic Lupus Erythematosus or Rheumatoid Arthritis. The outlook for patients with Non-Specific Pulmonary Fibrosis is also much better. 75% improve or stabilize on steroids and the mean survival is about 8 years, more than twice as long as UIP.

Hypersensitivity pneumonitis (HP) is due to an allergic reaction to inorganic and organic material such as proteins and bacteria. It is also known as "Extrinsic Allergic Alveolitis." It is an immunologically induced lung disease caused by repeated inhalation of a variety of environmental agents such as organic dusts and low molecular weight chemicals.

There are three stages of the disease. The acute stage occurs early in the course of the disease. About four to six hours after exposure to the offending agent, the patient develops fever, chills, cough and shortness of breath. If he goes to the emergency room, the chest radiograph will show a pattern similar to pulmonary edema or ARDS. Over the next few months during the subacute phase, with each subsequent exposure, the symptoms recur and linger longer. Finally, in the chronic phase, which develops over years, the patient has cough, shortness of breath, fever, and weight loss. The patient may or may not recall a history of acute episodes.

Hundreds of agents can cause the disease. The most common include "Farmer's Lung" due to a heat-loving bacteria known as Thermophilic actinomycetes, "Bird Fancier's Disease" due to protein droppings of budgerigars, pigeons, and even ducks, "Hot Tub Lung" due to Mycobacterium avium, "Bagassosis" due to exposure to sugar cane, and "Byssinosis" due to exposure to cotton. An organic chemical, Toluene diisocyanate, which has multiple uses including the making of computers can also cause the disease as can Pyrethrum which is an insecticide made from chrysanthemums.

The patient may have "Velcro rales" on the exam and, if the disease has been ongoing for some time, have significant weight loss.

In the chronic phase, the chest x-ray will show reticular infiltrates involving mainly the upper lobes. The high resolution CAT scan will show ground glass opacities which may be diffuse, patchy, or centrilobular in location associated with patchy areas of hyper-lucency due to focal areas of air trapping.

The biopsy will show bronchiolocentric interstitial pneumonitis associated with poorly formed interstitial granulomas as well as an organizing pneumonia.

The diagnosis is established in a patient with pulmonary fibrosis if the patient has a history of recurrent episodes of cough and shortness of breath occurring within four to eight hours of exposure to a known cause of the disease as well as positive precipitating antibodies to the causative agent.

The treatment is to avoid further exposure. Corticosteroids may or may not be helpful in the acute exposure. Once the chronic phase has developed, the disease tends to progress slowly.

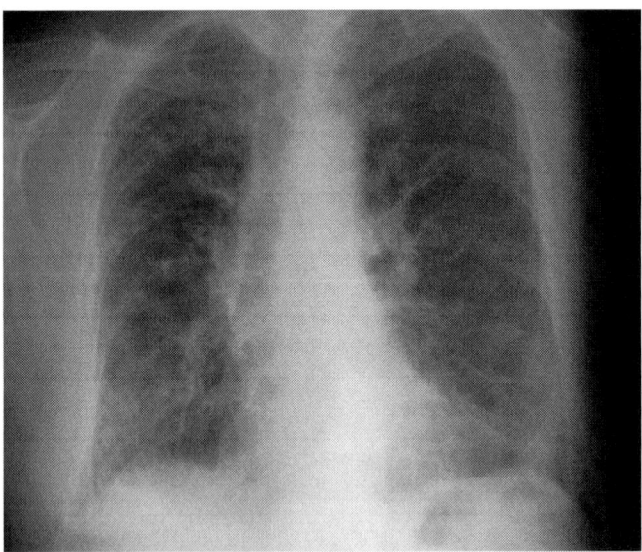

This is a patient with "Farmer's Lung". The chest x-ray shows a diffuse reticular infiltrate throughout the lungs but especially involving the upper lobes.

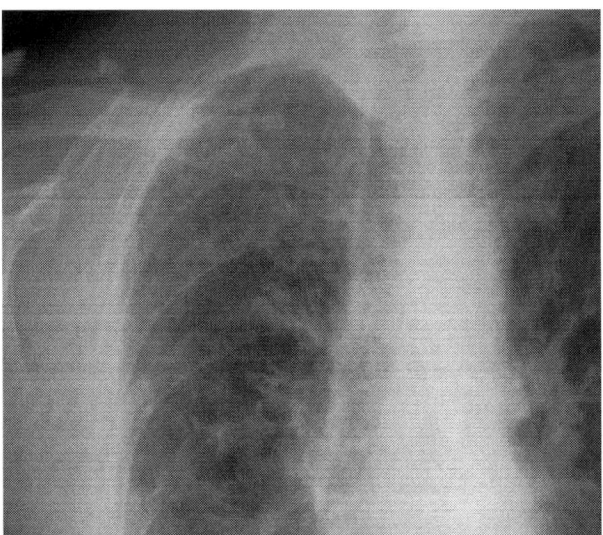

This is a close-up of the right upper lobe which is classic for "HP"

Sarcoidosis is an inflammatory disease characterized by the presence of innumerable tiny granulomas. The granulomas are nodules made up of swirls of fibrous tissue imbedded with multinucleated giant cells. In that sense they resemble the granulomas of tuberculosis. However, the center of the tubercular granulomas break down and form a cheesy or creamy center referred to as "caseous necrosis". This is NOT seen in Sarcoidosis. Sarcoid granulomas are "non-caseous granulomas."

Sarcoidosis is a multisystem disease. It involves not only the lungs, but also the eyes, heart and skin. In addition the patient often has systemic symptoms such as generalized weakness, fever, arthritis, weight loss and swollen lymph glands. Involvement of the heart leads to fatal arrhythmias. If the heart muscle is diseased, the patient may present with syncope (fainting), an irregular heartbeat or even signs of congestive heart failure. Eye symptoms include blurred vision, redness and pain in the eye and light sensitivity. The skin lesions are often characteristic and include red, painful nodules (erythema nodosum), sores on the nose, cheeks and ears (lupus pernio), as well as brownish patches of skin and nodules.

Most often, pulmonary sarcoidosis is asymptomatic. The disease is found on a routine chest x-ray. But the patient may also have shortness of breath, a dry cough, or even wheezing.

Sarcoidosis is in part genetic in that there are certain genes which govern the inflammatory pathway and make the patient more likely to get sarcoidosis given the right environment. If there is a family history of Sarcoidosis, there is definitely an increased risk of getting the disease. Health care workers, firefighters and people who work with insecticides are also more likely to get the disease. The disease is more common in Blacks as well as people of Scandinavian descent.

Sarcoidosis of the lung is divided into four stages:

Stage 1: The presence of large hilar lymph nodes on a chest radiograph. The hilar adenopathy is always bilateral. Unlike lymphomas which can also affect the hilar nodes, in Sarcoidosis there is a clear space between the right hilum and right heart border.

Stage 2: The presence of hilar adenopathy as well as interstitial changes in the lungs.

Stage 3: The presence of interstitial changes alone.

Stage 4: diffuse changes resembling emphysema.

The diagnosis is made by biopsy, usually through a bronchoscope. The lining of the trachea and a major airway is biopsied along with the lung. The presence of non-caseating granulomas is diagnostic.

The treatment of Sarcoidosis is multifactorial and is directed at the immune system. The first line of therapy is oral corticosteroids, including prednisone, in order to reduce inflammation. If there is no significant response, disease modifying agents, similar to the drugs used to treat rheumatoid arthritis, can be given. These include methotrexate, azathioprine, and leflunomide. If there is still no response, then infliximab, a monoclonal antibody, is used. Finally, corticotrophin or ACTH, which is the hormone that the pituitary secretes to stimulate the adrenal glands to produce cortisone, can be tried.

In general, if there is no evidence of pulmonary fibrosis, eye disease, heart disease or other critical organ involvement no treatment is given. Stage 1 disease of the lung should never be treated.

Pneumoconiosis

There are hundreds of occupations that can lead to lung disease. The two most studied are asbestosis and silicosis. Asbestosis causes a disease that looks like pulmonary fibrosis whereas silicosis causes myriad, sometimes extremely large, non-caseating granulomas, akin to Sarcoidosis.

Asbestosis is caused by the asbestos fiber which is shaped like a spear. It is very long and very thin. The fiber readily reaches the small airways where it impales the mucosa, penetrating into the pulmonary tissue. Some of the fibers even make their way to the pleural surface. The fiber is indestructible. It is heat resistant, acid resistant and chemical resistant. The pulmonary macrophages ingest the fiber but cannot destroy it. Over time some fibers disappear but most remain imbedded in the lung tissue, resulting in progressive interstitial fibrosis.

The fibers can also cause benign pleural disease called pleural plaques, lung cancers, cancers of the pleura called mesotheliomas, and even gastrointestinal cancers.

The list of "who gets asbestosis" is huge. It includes electricians, maintenance workers, iron workers and boilermakers, painters, carpenters, service station workers, body shop workers, and even oil field workers including roughnecks.

Symptoms include shortness of breath and cough. Physical findings include "Velcro Rales" as well as clubbing. Clubbing occurs late in the course of the disease. If you have a patient with asbestosis and clubbing, always look for a lung cancer.

The chest x-ray shows bibasilar interstitial changes which are generally reticular in type. The high resolution CAT scan will be diagnostic. There may also be calcified pleural plaques, which when combined with the interstitial changes are virtually diagnostic of the disease.

The pulmonary function studies may show obstructive disease early on in the course of the disease or restrictive disease with decreased diffusion later in the course of the disease.

The diagnosis is made clinically. There must be a history of significant exposure to the asbestos fiber, an adequate time for the disease to become manifest (ten years), and some sign of the disease such as shortness of breath or an abnormal chest x-ray. A biopsy is not needed.

There is no treatment. If the patient is young enough and sick enough, a lung transplant can be considered.

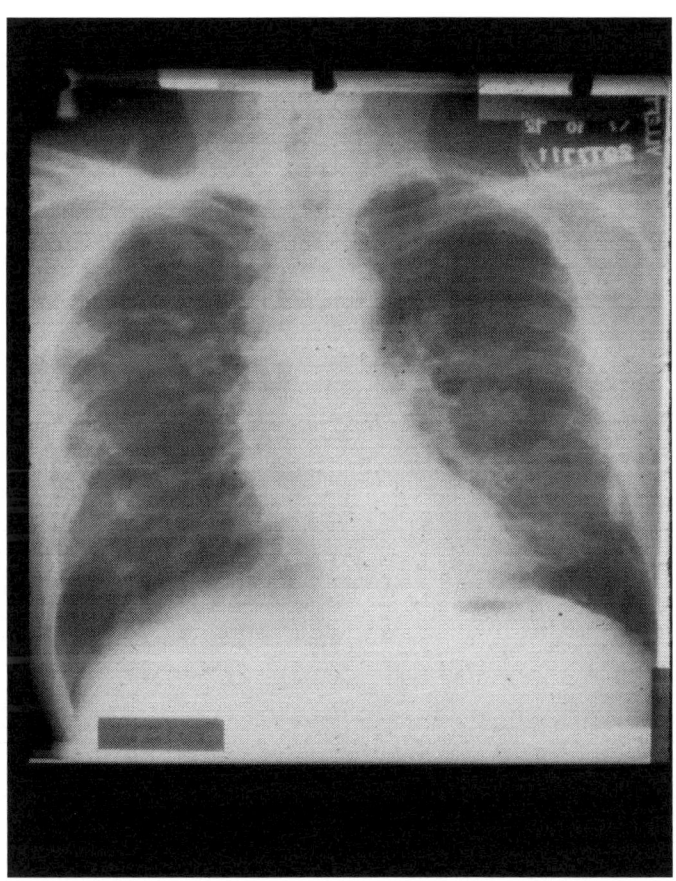

A patient with asbestosis and numerous calcified pleural plaques. The left heart border is obscured. This is called "The Shaggy Heart Sign".

Silicosis is an occupational lung disease due to the inhalation of quartz. It is characterized by the presence of the silicotic nodule. Silica or quartz particles have free radicals on their surface which cause an inflammatory reaction, but which are so potent that they overwhelm the body's defenses causing pulmonary fibrosis. Initially, the silica particles cause silicotic nodules to form around the small bronchioles as a collection of dust laden macrophages surrounded by a rim of fibrous tissue. The nodules gradually enlarge, growing at the periphery of the nodule, forming granulomas similar to the granuloma of Sarcoidosis. The growth of the nodules continues even after the exposure is ended. Ultimately progressive massive fibrosis is the result. This is a conglomeration of large nodules.

Silicosis is one of the oldest occupational disease. It is seen in miners, stone workers, abrasive workers, millers, glass makers, potters, and sandblasters.

There are two types of silicosis. The most common is chronic silicosis. It generally requires about 10 to 30 years of exposure to the silica particle. It may present as simple disease with minimal symptoms. The chest x-ray shows small rounded opacities in the upper lung fields associated with enlarged hilar lymph nodes. The pulmonary function testing is often normal. It may also present as massive pulmonary fibrosis. The patient has a cough, is dyspneic, and may go on to respiratory failure. The pulmonary function testing shows combined obstructive and restrictive disease.

Acute Silicosis is very rare. It is due to an exposure to an "overwhelming quantity of silica". The patient has a cough, weight loss and fatigue. The physical exam shows diffuse crackles as well as signs of right heart failure. The chest x-ray looks like pulmonary edema or ARDS and the disease progresses to death over a handful of months.

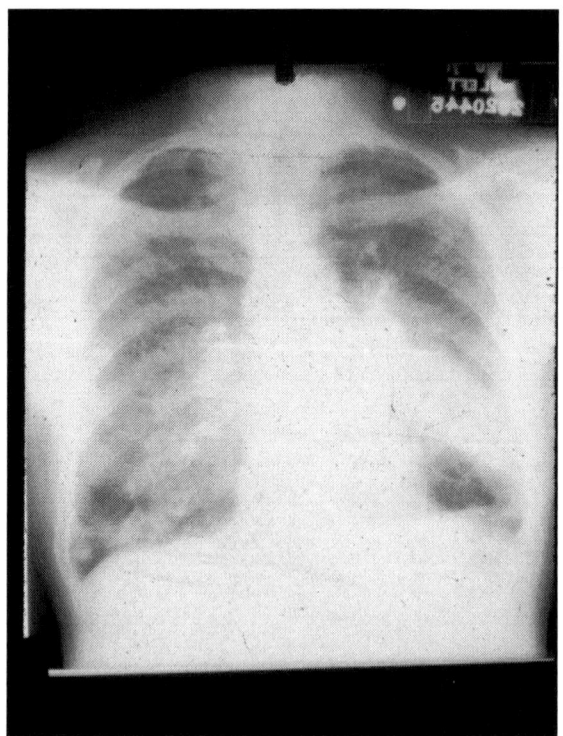

A patient with massive fibrosis with large masses of granulomas as well as diffuse interstitial changes.

In summary, the pulmonary function tests vary in the different types of restrictive diseases. In neuromuscular disease, because of muscle weakness, the total lung capacity is decreased and the residual volume is increased. But, unless there is some pulmonary fibrosis, the functional residual capacity and diffusion are normal. In obesity, because of the stiff chest wall, the total lung capacity, functional residual capacity and residual volume are all decreased but the diffusion is usually, though not necessarily, increased. In kyphoscoliosis because of muscle weakness the total lung capacity is decreased and the residual volume is increased. Because of the stiff chest wall the functional residual capacity is decreased. Diffusion is normal.

In contrast, in the interstitial lung disorders, the alveolar air is replaced by fluid, cellular infiltrates, or scar tissue. The lungs become stiff. Compliance is decreased and thus all the lung volumes are decreased. Diffusion is decreased as well.

IMPORTANT CONCEPTS TO REMEMBER FROM THIS LECTURE

1. Usual interstitial pneumonitis is characterized clinically by:

    Progressive shortness of breath associated with a dry cough in a middle-aged male, who on physical exam has "Velcro" crackles and may have clubbing and arthritis

2. Non-specific interstitial pneumonitis differs from UIP in that:

    It tends to occur in women as often in men in the 50's and is associated with a less honeycombing of the lung and more alveolar disease as seen by a ground glass appearance on HRCT. It responds to steroids and life expectancy is twice as long as UIP.

3. Farmer's lung is a type of:

    Hypersensitivity pneumonitis

4. Silicosis is characterized by:

    A progressive nodular disease, involving mainly the upper lobes, which ultimately results in massive fibrosis, shortness of breath, and death

5. If a patient has low lung volumes but an increased diffusion he or she most likely has:

    Morbid obesity

Chapter Eighteen

Sleep and Sleep Disorders

"Sleep no more. Macbeth doth murder sleep"

This famous line says a lot about sleep. Macbeth just killed Duncan, the king of Scotland, while he slept. For Macbeth sleep will no longer be peaceful and innocent. It will no longer be the nourisher and healer. But even more, if a king can be killed in his sleep, who among us is safe while we slumber?

Perhaps Sleep Apnea, Narcolepsy, and even the Restless Leg Syndrome are like Macbeth. They too murder sleep for millions and millions of people throughout the world.

But what is sleep? Sleep is defined as a naturally recurring state of suspended sensory and motor activity, characterized by near-total unconsciousness and the nearly complete inactivity of voluntary muscles, *from which the animal may be aroused easily by stimulation.*

Hibernation is characterized by a state of inactivity and metabolic depression resulting in marked lower body temperature, slower breathing and lower metabolic activity. *The creature cannot be awakened easily from this state.* The animal appears dead. There is no movement. The heart may beat only twice a minute.

While you are asleep, loud noises can wake you. You are arousable. In addition, you have spontaneous movements and your brain is active.

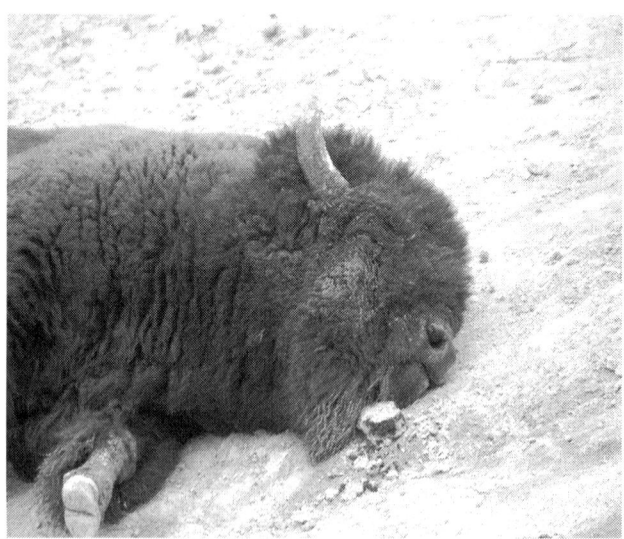

This little creature is only sleeping. Trust me! He is totally arousable!

Which animals sleep? All birds and mammals sleep as do most insects including the fruit fly. The lion sleeps 16 hours a day while his prey, the antelope, sleeps only seven. The bat sleeps 19 hours a day. Aquatic mammals such as seals and dolphins sleep with one side of their brain at a time. One eye is always open and one side of their brain is always awake.

Thus sleep is nearly ubiquitous. If so, why do we spend one third of our lives in a state of suspended animation? Several theories have been proposed.

1. **Adaptive**: sleeping at night keeps us out of harm's way. Not likely. Predators sleep far more than their prey!

2. **Energy conservation**: The sleeping animal uses 15% less energy. His temperature falls up to 2 degrees. But this is not likely either. The cost of sleeping is the increased risk of becoming someone else's dinner.

3. **Restorative function**: Growth hormone increases at night resulting in improved immune system functioning and muscle growth. Brain Adenosine, derived from ATP and cyclic AMP, builds up in the brain during the day and must be resynthesized into ATP at night. Increased levels of Adenosine increase deep sleep. Caffeine is an adenosine antagonist and keeps us awake. Sleep deprivation increases levels of adenosine.

4. **Brain Plasticity**: While we are asleep the brain organizes what has happened throughout the day resulting in better learning.

Studies have shown that restoring our body and brain function as well as learning are the main reasons we sleep. The brain is only 2% of body mass by weight but it uses 20% of the body's metabolism. The brain can use only glucose (fats and proteins are not available) for energy production. The brain requires a lot of ATP which is broken down into adenosine. The adenosine increases the movement of potassium in the potassium channel which hyperpolarizes the neuron allowing the calcium channel to "deinactivate" resulting in deep sleep. The more intense the brain activity during the day, the longer the deep sleep.

The evidence for the importance of sleep in improving learning is compelling. There are two types of sleep, non-REM and REM sleep. Non-REM sleep is everything from drowsiness to deep sleep. REM sleep is Rapid Eye Movement sleep. During REM sleep, the brain appears to be awake but the body is paralyzed except for the eye muscles and diaphragm. The EEG of rats working a maze during the day is repeated at night during REM sleep. Learned physical tasks, such as typing a particular pattern on a computer keyboard, are performed better after a restful sleep. Word-pairs are remembered better after sleep. There is increased insight after sleeping. Learning is enhanced after an afternoon nap if it includes both non-REM and REM sleep. Both non-REM and REM sleep are required for memory and learning.

Learning is a two-step process. We must first encode the event, turning the event into a memory and thus into a particular sequence of neuronal activity. Then we must consolidate the memory by strengthening the new neuronal pathway, and associating it with similar pathways already present in the brain. Then we must transfer the event and pathway to long term memory while we erase memories we no longer need.

There is a fast and a slow component to making a memory. The fast component occurs in non-REM sleep. The center for this activity is found in the *hippocampus*. The hippocampus relates new events to old memories and packages the new and the old memories together. It then sends the "package" to the cerebral cortex where, during REM sleep, the old and new memories are integrated.

The hippocampus is the memory center. Without this part of the brain you can't make memories. The hippocampus is very large in taxi drivers in London. The more experienced the taxi drivers, the larger the hippocampi. Taxi drivers in London require a lot of memory because they are required by law, if they want to get their license, to know where every street in that ancient city is located. When I was in medical school I was taught that you never make more neurons. What you have when you are born is all you are going to get. That is simply not true. Neurogenesis is occurring daily in the hippocampus, but the survival of the new cells depends in part upon getting a good night's sleep!

Even things like playing tennis or playing the piano are helped by sleep. Learning a new task involves repetition of the task. But if we practice the task in the morning, by late afternoon we don't do quite as well. However, after a good night's sleep we do the task 20% better and the improvement will continue for up to five days, so long as we get a decent sleep those five days.

Thus sleep is very important for us! But how much sleep do we need? Newborn and Infants need to sleep about 16 hours a day of which half is REM sleep, while young children sleep about 9 hours a day as REM sleep slowly decreases. At puberty, the amount of REM sleep has decreased to about 30% of the total sleep time. In addition, the onset of sleep is delayed. "Larks become Owls." The fully mature adult requires about 8 hours of sleep of which 20-25% is REM sleep. Every decade after middle age requires about 20 minutes less sleep so that patients over 70 require between 5 and 6 ½ hours of sleep. Sleeping less than 5 hours or more than 7 hours is associated with illness. After 70, REM accounts for only about 20-25% of sleep time and sleep becomes more and more fragmented.

What determines how much sleep we need? The longer we are awake, the more non-REM sleep we need. The more non-REM sleep we have, the more REM sleep we need to get. The more sleep deprived we are, the longer we will be in delta or Stage 3 non-REM sleep. We must pay back our sleep debt.

What other factors affect our sleep? In addition to age, sleep is difficult if the patient has an illness with fever, or has pain, or is under stress. Even sleeping in a room with too much light, especially the blue light of a cell phone, or a noisy room, or a room that is too hot, will make it much more difficult to get a good sleep. Severe fatigue will decrease the amount of our REM sleep. Alcohol will make us sleepy but will fragment our sleep. Chemicals such as antihistamines and nicotine have the same effect. Loosing or gaining weight also affects sleep. Weight loss leads to more arousals and decreased sleep time while weight gain increases total sleep time and decreases arousals.

How long can we go without sleep? In 1964, Randy Gardner, who was sixteen at the time, set the scientifically documented record for the longest period of time a human being has intentionally gone without sleep not using stimulants of any kind. Gardner stayed awake for 264 hours (11 days). Lt. Cmdr. John J. Ross, who monitored his health, reported serious cognitive and behavioral changes which included moodiness, problems with concentration and short term memory, paranoia and hallucinations. However, on his final day, Gardner gave a press conference where he spoke clearly and appeared to be in good health. That evening he went to bed and slept 14 hours and then the next day slept 10 hours. He appeared to be in good health afterwards.

The previous record was held by Peter Tripp, a DJ, which he set in 1959. He did a "wake-a-thon" for a charity. By the fourth day he began having delusions. He saw spiders in his shoes! He ultimately made 201 hours. He slept for 20 hours but afterwards had psychotic problems. His marriage broke up and he lost his job. He ended up selling books door to door.

There are several known effects of sleep deprivation including confusion, memory lapses, depression, development of false memories, hallucinations, hand tremor, headaches, malaise, periorbital puffiness, commonly known as "bags under the eyes" and increased blood pressure. More serious side effects include increased stress hormone levels, increased risk of diabetes, irritability, nystagmus (rapid involuntary rhythmic eye movement), seizures, temper tantrums in children, mania, symptoms similar to attention-deficit hyperactivity disorder (ADHD) and psychosis.

A recent study of 4,000 adults showed that getting less than six hours of sleep a night is quite harmful. The study was reported in October of 2018 by Dr. Fernando Dominquez at the European Society of Cardiology annual meeting. The patients with less than six hours of sleep a night were more likely to be overweight, have a higher blood pressure, and suffer from the metabolic syndrome. They also had more atherosclerosis.

Anatomy of Sleep

There are several parts of the brain that are important in the sleep-wake cycle. The Reticular Activating System, located in the upper brainstem, is important in waking us up. If the RAS is diseased we will sleep forever, even though the cerebral cortex is normal.

Between 1915 and 1926 there was an epidemic of encephalitis lethargica which affected more than 5 million people. It is a form of encephalitis commonly referred to as "sleeping sickness." It was first described by the neurologist Constantin von Economo in 1917. It appears to be an autoimmune disease and initially was thought to be related to the great flu epidemic that spanned the world at the time. More recent evidence suggests that the disease was related to Streptococcal pharyngitis. The disease attacks the RAS leaving the patient in a statue-like condition. The patient sits motionless, speechless, totally lacking in initiative, appetite, affect or desire. Whatever happens around him does not affect him in the slightest. One scientist described the patients as ghosts or zombies. About one third of the patients died. None recovered fully.

The hypothalamus also is important in wakefulness. It secretes *hypocretin* which promotes wakefulness, helps maintain motor control and inhibits REM sleep during wakefulness.

On the other hand the anterior hypothalamus is involved in making us sleepy. It receives input from the body's "clock", the suprachiasmatic nucleus. The neurotransmitter is Gabapentin, which turns off the centers for wakefulness. If the hypothalamus fails, the patient will stay awake till he drops dead. The condition is called Fatal Familial Insomnia which is a prion disease like Mad Cow's Disease. Fatal Familial Insomnia can either be genetic or, less commonly, sporadic. The gene, an autosomal dominant, is found in no more than forty families worldwide. The disease presents in middle age as progressively worsening insomnia, leading to hallucinations, delirium, dementia, and eventually, death, usually within eighteen months of the onset of symptoms. The first recorded case was an Italian man, who died in Venice in 1765.

The center for REM sleep is in the Pons. Lesions below the pons result in EEG findings consistent with REM sleep in the cortex but no muscle atonia while lesions above the pons shows no cortical changes of REM sleep, but muscle atonia. The neurotransmitter is acetyl choline which "wakes up" the cerebral cortex. If acetyl choline is decreased by damaging the Pons, REM sleep decreases. Acetyl choline analogs injected into the Pons increase REM sleep.

Sleep Architecture

Sleep is divided into two stages, non-REM and REM sleep. Non-REM sleep is further divided into three stages, stage 1 which is light sleep, stage 2 which is the predominant stage of sleep, and stage 3 which is deep sleep. Each stage is characterized by the type of brain waves observed and the clinical state of the patient. In general there are four types of brain waves. Alpha waves are slightly large and fast. They are generally seen when we are in light sleep. Beta waves are smaller and faster still. They are found in when we are awake or are just a little drowsy. Theta waves are larger and slower waves and are found in stage two sleep. Delta waves are the slowest and largest wave. They are seen in deep sleep.

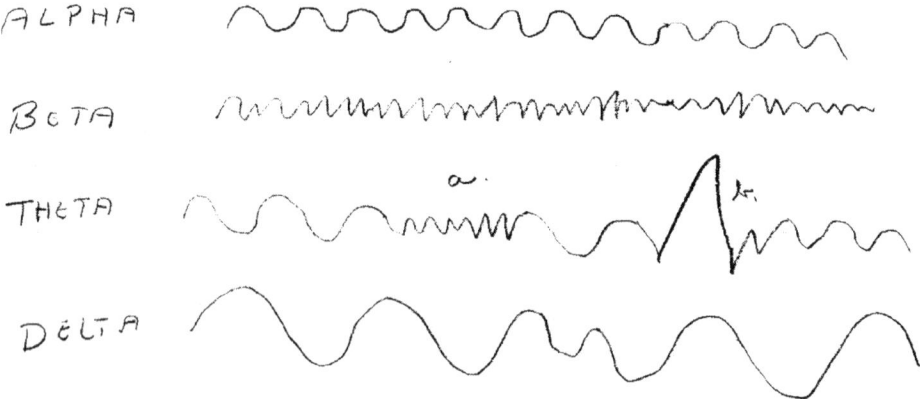

The graph compares the different types of waves found during sleep. The "a" is a sleep spindle while "b" is a K complex.

Stage one or light sleep is characterized by the presence of alpha and beta waves. As the person falls into stage one sleep he or she may experience a sudden generalized muscle jerk which is called a Hypnic Myoclonia. It is totally normal. In stage one, the eyes may show slow, rolling movements. There is decreased muscle activity. The heart rate, blood pressure, minute ventilation and cerebral blood flow are all decreased. If the patient is aroused, he will say he hasn't been sleeping at all even though he may have been snoring!

Stage two is the predominant type of sleep. It accounts for 40-50% of sleep. The EEG shows slow theta waves which are interrupted by bursts of large waves called sleep spindles and K complexes. These complexes are due to communication between the cerebral cortex and the thalamus or hippocampus. They are likely related to learning. There may also be slow rolling eye motion or the eyes may be fixed. The muscles are relaxed. The patient is easily arousable but snoring is often present.

Stage three or deep sleep is characterized by the presence of high amplitude delta waves. The muscles are inactive and there is no eye movement. The pulse rate, blood pressure and respiratory rate are all 30% below levels found when we are awake. The patient may dream but the dreams are not bizarre. Bed-wetting and sleep-walking may occur.

REM sleep is a complete contrast to non-REM sleep. The first episode of REM sleep occurs about 90 minutes after falling asleep and recurs about every 90 minutes afterwards. Most of the REM sleep occurs in the second half of sleep. The main feature is the presence of rapid eye movement and alpha waves. The EEG appears similar to when the patient is awake! However, all the muscles, except for the diaphragm and the eye muscles are paralyzed. The heart rate and blood pressure increase. During this phase the patient often has vivid, bizarre dreams.

Throughout the night the patient cycles between the stages of sleep. A graph of the cycling is called a hypnogram. The brain goes from awake to drowsy to Stage 1 NREM, then Stage 2 NREM, then Stage 3 NREM sleep before going into REM. It then recycles another four times during the night, roughly every 90 minutes, until finally the patient awakens, generally, from an episode of REM sleep. The length of the sleep cycle in animals and man is related to the size of the brain.

How do we study sleep? A **polysomnogram** is a sleep study. It can be done in the sleep laboratory (Level 1 Sleep Study). During the study we measure several parameters including the electroencephalogram (EEG) to determine the level of sleep, the electroculogram (EOG) to look at eye movements in order to separate non-REM from REM sleep, the electromyogram (EMG) to study muscle tone, the EKG to look at heart rate and the presence of cardiac arrhythmias, and impedance plethysmography of the chest wall and abdomen to look at respiration in order to determine the presence of air flow and movement of the abdominal and chest wall. The sleep study can also be done at home (Level 3 sleep study) when only a nasal cannula, pulse oximeter, and a device to measure respiratory effort are used. Since an EEG is not done, the AHI can't be measured—only the incidence of events occurring over the whole course of the study whether the patient is asleep or awake. Thus, the frequency of apneas and hypopneas will be significantly underestimated.

Students have the most difficulty understanding impedance plethysmography. Air flow can only occur due to movement of the respiratory muscles of the chest or respiratory muscles of the abdomen or both. If the airway is blocked, the chest wall will suck in while the abdomen expands or the abdomen will suck in while the chest wall expands. The sum of the movements of the chest wall and abdomen will be zero.

Impedance is the resistance to the flow of alternating current.

Voltage = Current X Impedance

When the voltage is constant an increase in the impedance will cause a fall in the current or flow of electrons. If we place a series of coils close together in an alternating current circuit the negative charges of the electrons will repel each other and increase the impedance and thus decrease the current flow. When the coils are spread apart the electrons can move better and impedance falls. The current flow increases.

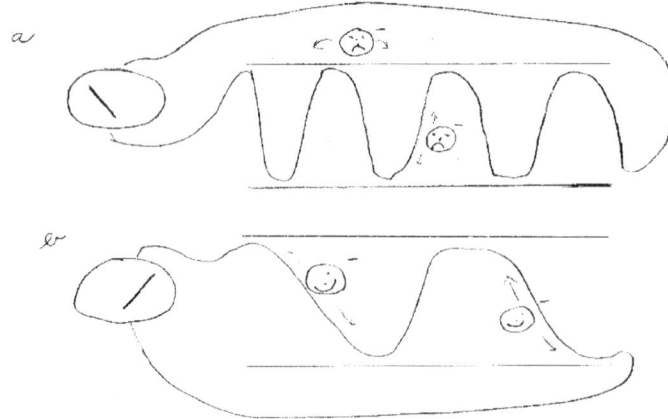

In a, the coils are close together. The electrons are unhappy because they have little freedom of movement and the current is low. In b, the coils are farther apart. The electrons are happy because they have more freedom and can move easily. The current is faster.

Thus we can determine if there is normal air movement or apnea by placing one impedance belt around the chest and one around the abdomen and then studying the resulting tracings.

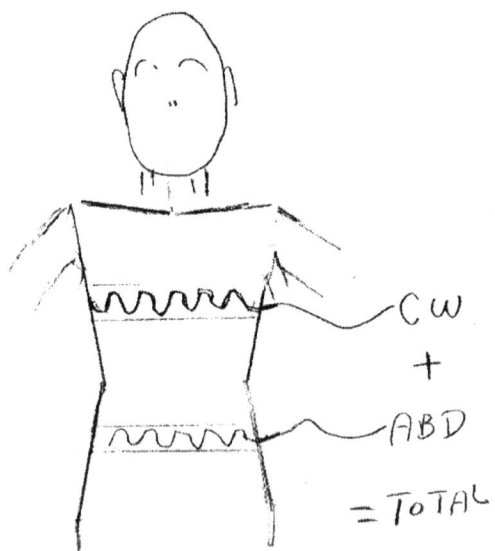

One coil is placed around the chest wall and one around the abdomen. If the coils are placed correctly and calibrated, the total volume will equal the chest volume plus the abdominal volume.

The normal patient will show that the abdominal and thoracic component move in the same direction during quiet breathing while the patient with obstructive sleep apnea will show the abdominal and thoracic components moving in opposite directions during apneas and hypopneas while the patient with central sleep apnea won't have any abdominal or thoracic movement at all during apneas.

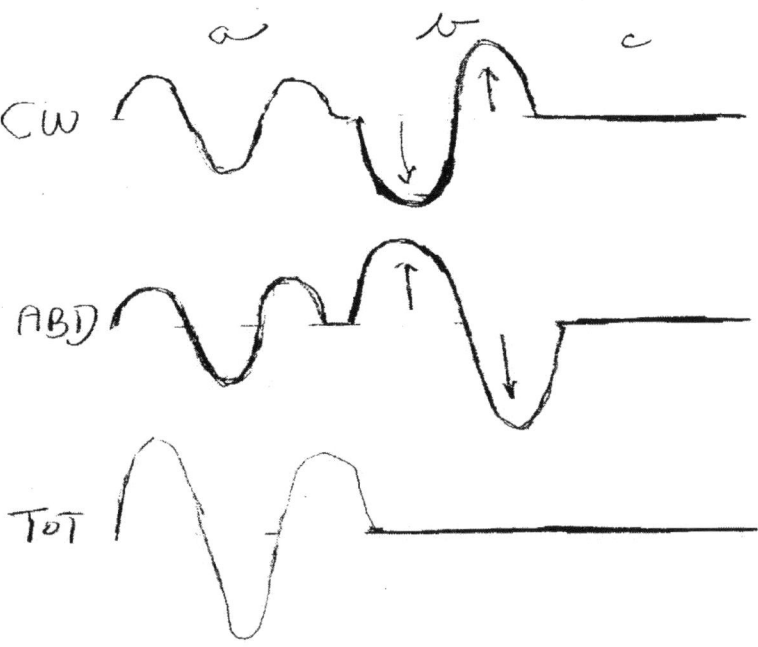

A continuous tracing of the Impedance Plethysmography of the chest wall (CW), abdomen (ABD), and total (TOT). In (a) chest wall and abdominal wall movement are in the same direction and the total movement or air flow is the sum of the two volumes. In (b) there is no airflow. The total volume change is zero. But there is respiratory effort as shown by the CW and ABD moving in equal and opposite directions. The patient is clearly obstructed. In (c) there is no air movement as again. TOT is zero. But now there is no abdominal wall or chest wall change either. The patient has central apnea.

Surprisingly impedance plethysmography is as accurate as spirometry in measuring the vital capacity when it is calibrated correctly.

Sleep Disorders

Sleep disorders can be divided into two large groups. The most common is insomnia or the perceived inability to sleep. The second group is those people who are always sleepy.

Insomnia is never a diagnosis. It is a symptom. It is defined as difficulty initiating or maintaining sleep or both. Recurrent insomnia affects up to 50% of people, but 95% of people report having had at least one episode of insomnia in their life and ten percent have chronic insomnia. Chronic insomnia occurs more often in women and its frequency increases as we age.

Certain factors make insomnia worse. It is aggravated by over activity and stress which may be related to man's ability to suppress sleep during stress. During 'on-call' nights doctors have disrupted sleep, even if they are not called. Insomnia, even transient insomnia, causes sleep deprivation resulting in daytime fatigue and impaired cognition, both of which can have serious complications.

Transient insomnia is insomnia that *lasts less than two weeks*. It is generally caused by one of three things. It can be due to hyper-alertness which is related to stress, either good or bad. It can also be due to changing Time Zones or performing Shift Work as in a couple who takes a vacation to Europe or in fireman who has constant changes in his or her work hours. Lastly environmental factors such as loud noises and bright lights can play a role. Of interest, the blue light from our cell phones is often a cause of insomnia.

Persistent insomnia is more of a problem. It is defined as insomnia lasting more than two weeks. It can be caused by:

Problems with the biologic clock—circadian rhythm.

Hyperthyroidism.

Hypercorticism including treatment with prednisone.

Restless Leg Syndrome and periodic limb movement disorder.

Gastroesophageal Reflux

Fibromyalgia.

Psychological disease including phobias, anxiety and depression

Primary Insomnia.

Sleep State Misperception

Most of the conditions above are self-explanatory but Fibromyalgia, primary insomnia and sleep-state misperception need more explanation.

Fibromyalgia is a disease of unknown etiology. The symptoms are vague and include muscle pain and weakness which is associated with tender areas on several parts of the body as well as general fatigue. Insomnia plays a large role in the symptomatology. While these patients have daytime fatigue their sleep latency is normal. The EEG is abnormal with alpha waves superimposed on delta waves.

Primary Insomnia has its onset in childhood. It is disorder of the brain mechanism that controls sleeping and waking. It is often associated with anxiety and tension. If the onset occurs in later years the patient states that he or she sleeps better away from home than at home. Clinically there should be symptoms of sleep deprivation and a prolonged sleep latency.

The last disorder is those patients with *sleep state misperception*. They really believe they do not sleep but when tested in the sleep lab, their sleep is totally normal. In addition, multiple sleep latency testing is normal indicating there isn't any daytime sleepiness. Thus they believe they are unable to sleep but their "sleeplessness" never affects their daytime functioning.

Daytime hypersomnolence is a "horse of a different color." There are three main causes: sleep apnea, either obstructive sleep apnea or central sleep apnea, narcolepsy and the restless leg syndrome.

What are apneas? We all stop breathing while we are asleep once in a while but it is uncommon. In fact, in normal people apneas occurs less than five times an hour. An apnea is when we stop breathing. For the apnea to be significant it must be more than 10 seconds long. Patients with **obstructive sleep apnea** stop breathing because their airway becomes blocked. This is almost always due to the anterior pharyngeal wall falling back against the posterior wall during an inspiration. The patient still makes the effort to breath but just can't move any air. In contrast people with **central sleep apnea** stop making the effort to breathe. The brain stops sending the signal to the muscles to breathe. There is no respiratory effort at all.

Sometimes the patient doesn't breathe as deeply as normal. A **hypopnea** is defined as an episode of breathing in which the tidal breath is reduced 30% and the oxygen saturation falls at least 4%. A third type of disturbed sleep is **respiratory effort related arousals**. These are episodes in which the patient arouses from sleep without meeting the criteria for either an apneic or hypopneic event.

Obstructive Sleep Apnea (OSA) is the most common cause of daytime sleepiness. The first description of a patient with the condition was by the writer Charles Dickens in the 19th century. In his book *The Pickwick Papers* he described a young man, a waiter at the Pickwick Club, named "Little Joe," who was extremely obese and suffered from severe daytime sleepiness. Little Joe even fell asleep while standing and knocking on the door of a member of the Pickwick Club.

The hallmark of the disorder is daytime sleepiness associated with significant apneic events occurring while asleep. The patient or the significant other often reports snoring and startles which are described as "waking up choking". After the patient falls asleep he will begin having episodes of obstructed breathing. During an episode, air flow will stop, but the patient will continue to move his chest wall and abdominal muscles as if he is gasping for air. After anywhere from ten seconds to a minute and a half, he will suddenly gasp or sit up and gasp. Then, he will lay back down and fall asleep, only to start the cycle over again.

The incidence of OSA is generally reported to be about 4% of men and 2% of women. These numbers were obtained in the early 1990's when the percentage of obese citizens in every state in the USA was less than 20%. Now, the percentage of obese citizens is more than 20% in every state and more than 30% in most states. Thus, the USA is much more obese now than it was 30 years ago. Because of that, the incidence of mild OSA (an AHI of > 5) is now 20-30% in men and 10-20% in women. If the bar for diagnosing sleep apnea is set at moderate OSA with an AHI of > 15, the incidence is 15% of men and 5% of women. But after a woman passes menopause she has the same chance of having OSA as a similarly aged man..

The patients with obstructive sleep apnea are often obese with a large neck size (greater than 17.5) and a waist size greater than 38. They also tend to be older and are more often men. They may have chronic nasal congestion. Smoking, alcohol abuse, and some classes of medication especially Beta blockers and antihistamines, will worsen the condition. Blacks, Hispanics, and Pacific Islanders are more likely to have obstructive sleep apnea than Whites.

The condition is also seen in patients with craniofacial abnormalities such as micrognathia, or in patients with Hypothyroidism, Acromegaly, Down's syndrome or large tonsil's (children and patients with HIV). Lastly it can occur in familial aggregations. These patients are often normal in weight and younger than the typical patient.

Surprisingly Asians have the same incidence of sleep apnea as Americans even though they are much less likely to be overweight. Likely this is related to cranial-facial differences, primarily a small mid face.

The first step in making the diagnosis is to determine if the patient has daytime sleepiness. The easiest test to determine this is the Epworth Sleepiness Scale. The patient is asked the likelihood that he or she will fall asleep during certain activities.

Activity	Score
Sitting and reading	* (0, 1, 2, or 3)
Watching TV	
Sitting inactive in a public place	
Passenger in a car	
Lying down to rest in the afternoon	
Sitting talking to someone	
Sitting after a lunch without alcohol	
In a car stopped in traffic for a few minutes	
TOTAL SCORE (normal is less than 10)	

* = (0 = never, 1 = slight chance, 2 = moderate chance, 3 = high chance)

If the patient has daytime hypersomnolence then a sleep study should be conducted. The number of apneas and hypopneas should be measured. Each episode must last 10 seconds and a hypopnea must be associated with a significant fall in tidal volume and oxygen saturation. The sum of the apneas and hypopneas is expressed as the A-H index (AHI) which is simply the number of these events per hour of sleep. Normal is less than 5. Mild sleep apnea is 5-15; moderate sleep apnea is 15-30 and severe obstructive sleep apnea is more than 30 events an hour. Some apneas can last more than a minute!

Another study which can also be done to evaluate daytime sleepiness is the multiple sleep latency test (MSLT). This test consists of having the patient take five naps at two hour intervals during the day, often the day following the overnight sleep study. The patient is asked to lie quietly and try to sleep. Each test is done for up to 20 minutes. Sleep latency is the time from lights out to first epoch of sleep lasting more than 15 seconds during a 30 second period. Average latencies of less than five minutes are abnormal. If REM sleep occurs during the MSLT, a condition called narcolepsy is very likely. We will discuss narcolepsy shortly.

The treatment of obstructive sleep apnea includes positive pressure breathing either with a CPAP or a BIPAP device. Both these devices apply positive pressure through the nasal or oral pharynx in order to keep the airway open throughout inspiration and expiration. If that fails to stop the obstruction a tracheostomy will be curative. Many people don't like having to use the positive pressure device and nobody ever wants a tracheostomy. Often the patient will elect to have surgery including radiofrequency ablation of the fatty tissue at the back of the throat or a UPPP (Uvulopalatopharyngoplasty) in which the tonsils and adenoids are removed and the uvula, soft palate, and pharynx are modified. These less invasive surgeries are not effective. Dental appliances work only for the mildest cases. A newer surgical approach involves electrical stimulation of the hypoglossal nerve which draws the anterior pharynx anteriorly and opens the airway. A sensor evaluates muscle activity in the chest wall. When activity is noted, a signal is sent to stimulate the hypoglossal nerve to contract and the airway is opened. This type of therapy is likely to become a standard therapy but the surgery is quite costly.

The most effective surgery involves maxillary-mandibular advancement which is quite invasive but has an 80-90% success rate.

The long term effects of untreated sleep apnea are severe and include both *Alzheimer's disease* and the *Metabolic Syndrome*. Sleep apnea is the second most common treatable cause of Alzheimer's disease. The most common treatable cause is hypertension. About half of patients with Alzheimer's disease have sleep-disordered breathing. Sleep apnea causes hypoxemia which damages brain cells. There is a growing body of evidence to support this hypothesis. One study showed that rats exposed for 16 hours a day to decreased O2 levels developed plaques in the brain similar to those of patients with Alzheimer's disease. Another study showed that patients with sleep apnea have "shrunken brain structures" in the part of the brain associated with memory. A third study using a very sensitive MRI study of the brain showed scattered areas (prefrontal, parietal and temporal) of brain damage in patients with sleep apnea.

Even patients with obstructive sleep apnea who are asymptomatic have recently been shown to have problems with recent memory. But in contrast to Alzheimer's disease who have worse memories at 30 minutes compared to 5 minutes, patients with obstructive sleep apnea have worse recall at 5 minutes compared to 30 minutes.[5]

Another complication of sleep apnea is the Metabolic Syndrome. The Metabolic Syndrome is defined as the development of insulin resistance resulting in central obesity, diabetes, hypertension and hyperlipidemia. It is caused by the release of inflammatory chemicals such as tumor necrotic factor from the fatty tissue which causes plaques in arteries of the heart, the brain and other tissues. Kono et al studied NON-obese patients with OSA and found that hyperglycemia and hypertension were more common in patients with OSA than in matched controls and the abnormalities were directly related to the AHI. Still another study showed that TIA's and strokes were associated significantly with sleep apnea. Lastly, treatment with CPAP improves insulin sensitivity in patients with OSA. In one study, glucose levels improved significantly after three months of CPAP therapy.

If the metabolic syndrome wasn't enough, sleep apnea is also associated with depression, suicide, auto accidents, impaired performance at work and even an increased risk of infection due to decreased immune function.

---

[5] Dexter, DD, Ebert AG, A Unique Pattern on Memory Testing in Dementia Screening predicts Obstructive Sleep Apnea. WMJ 2019, 118 (1) 27-29

Central sleep apnea is very uncommon. The brain fails to send a signal to the respiratory muscles to contract. It is generally seen in patients who have significantly impaired neurologic disease as well as cardiac disease. These patients develop Cheyne-Stokes respiration which is a waxing and waning of respiration ending in an apneic episode. Central apnea is also associated with narcotic use and may occur at high altitude. It is also seen in patients with left ventricular failure, stroke and atrial fibrillation. Treatment currently involves using a non-invasive ventilator such as BIPAP. Neuro-stimulation may become an alternative therapy in the future. In fact, phrenic nerve stimulation is now FDA approved for the treatment of central sleep apnea. In one study, the AHI was cut in half and the arousals were decreased 80% with phrenic nerve stimulation. More than 90% of the patients had no ill effects from the treatment.

Narcolepsy is an uncommon cause of daytime hypersomnolence but it certainly is quite interesting. The term Narcolepsy is from the Greek and means "stupor attack". It is defined as *"Sleep-Wake State Instability"*. It is "an awake brain inside a sleeping body." For an unexplained reason the physiology of sleep intrudes into wakefulness. Classic Narcolepsy or Narcolepsy Type 1 is characterized not only by daytime sleepiness but also by **Cataplexy** as well as early onset REM sleep. Narcolepsy Type 2 differs in that there is no cataplexy. In both forms the patient often describes bizarre hallucinations at the onset of sleep. Lastly the patient may have sleep paralysis, during which, as he or she begins to fall asleep, he or she becomes paralyzed. The paralysis only lasts a very short period of time but is none the less quite frightening.

Cataplexy is muscle weakness which occurs whenever the patients gets excited. It may involve weakness in the facial muscles, the legs or the arms or the patient may just totally collapse. It can last just a few seconds or several minutes.

Narcolepsy can have its onset at any age. The incidence is about 1 in every 2000 people or about 250,000 people world-wide. It is, at least in part, a genetic disease though inheritance is limited. If you have narcolepsy, there is a 1% chance that your child will also have the disease. Most cases of narcolepsy appear to be sporadic. The onset of the disease is usually in the mid-teens or in the early twenties and thirties. Some animals, especially goats and dachshunds can be affected as well as humans.

The diagnosis is made during the sleep study. REM sleep normally does not occur until more than 45 minutes into sleep. In patients with Narcolepsy REM sleep occurs within eight minutes of falling asleep and is associated with "hypnagogic hallucinations" or night terrors which are severe, vivid nightmares which occur at the onset of sleep. Unlike patients with schizophrenia, patients with narcolepsy do NOT hear voices and they are aware that these "terrors" are not real.

If the sleep study is not diagnostic then a multiple sleep latency test should be done. The diagnosis is established if, in two of the naps during the study, REM sleep occurs within eight minutes of napping.

Narcolepsy is an auto-immune disorder which attacks cells of the hypothalamus which produces the chemical hypocretin. Hypocretin increases appetite and produces wakefulness. Hypocretin receptors are found in wake-promoting regions of the brain. In patients with Type 1 Narcolepsy, hypocretin levels are immeasurable in the CSF and hypocretin staining cells are absent in the hypothalamus.

Narcolepsy results in poor school and work performance because of daytime sleepiness. In addition it also causes social impairment (avoiding social activities) because of fear of a cataplexic attack. Both these effects lead to isolation and alienation.

The treatment of narcolepsy is at best only fair. Stimulants such as Ritalin or Provigil (a pseudo-amphetamine) are used to keep the patient awake. Anti-cataplectic agents including the antidepressants Imipramine and Prozac (SSRI) are also used. The newest and the most effective agent is Zyrem or sodium oxybate which is a central nervous system depressant. It helps prevent cataplexy as well as improve daytime sleepiness.

A simple "non-drug" therapy is the use of scheduled naps of 15-20 minutes. The naps will improve daytime wakefulness. Coffee can be used as well. Medications which can cause sedation, such as certain antihistamines such as Benadryl, should be avoided.

People with narcolepsy should not sit for a prolonged time at school or at work and should never work as long-haul truck drivers.

Periodic Leg Movement (PLM) is a common cause of daytime sleepiness. It is characterized by the involuntary twitching or jerking movements occurring while the patient is asleep. It can begin at any age but worsens with aging. Women tend to be more affected than men. While there is some evidence that it may be in part genetic, medications such as Haldol, Reglan, antihistamines, SSRI antidepressants such as Prozac, and alcohol definitely can cause it. It is often associated with the **restless leg syndrome (RSL)**. This syndrome occurs during the day, usually in the evening. The person's legs seem to want to move all the time. They burn or itch. The patient feels like there is something crawling under their skin. If the person tries to keep the legs still, the symptoms get worse. If the patient gets up and moves about, the symptoms are relieved for a short time. About 80% of patients with restless leg syndrome have the periodic leg movement disorder.

The initial treatment is to improve the lifestyle of the patient. Iron deficiency can cause the disorder. Check for Iron deficiency and treat it if it is present. Cut out alcohol, caffeine and tobacco. A sleep study should be done because both PLM and RLS are associated with obstructive sleep apnea and treating the sleep apnea can eliminate the PLM.

Medications can be helpful but often have more side effects than benefits. Dopaminergic agents such as Requip are the first line of therapy but long term use leads to worsening of the condition and the drug can cause obsessive behavior such as shopping as well as nausea and dizziness. Another drug is Gabapentin which works on the central nervous system and promotes sleep. Lastly short acting Benzodiazepines such as Klonopin can be tried. These drugs are addicting and should be avoided if possible.

IMPORTANT CONCEPTS TO REMEMBER FROM THIS LECTURE

1. Sleep differs from hibernation because:

    During hibernation the animal shows a marked decrease in metabolism resulting in a temperature often near the environmental temperature as well as difficulty in arousal from the state. With sleep the animal is readily arousable.

2. Which stage of sleep is most predominant?

    Stage two

3. Obstructive sleep apnea is characterized by:

    Absent flow rates associated with paradoxical movement of the abdominal and chest wall

4. The most common sleep disorder is:

    Insomnia

5. Narcolepsy is characterized by:

    Early onset REM sleep, daytime sleepiness, nightmares on falling asleep and cataplexy

6. Sleep is needed for:

    Learning and restoration of brain function

Chapter Nineteen

Anatomy and Physiology of the Kidneys

Part One: the Kidney

Anatomy

The kidneys are certainly underappreciated. When a young man breaks off a relationship with a beautiful young lady, no one ever speaks about a "broken kidney". Likewise, when someone dies they are never said to have "taken their last pee." No, the kidneys are truly unloved. Yet without the kidneys, the heart, lungs and brain would be totally functionless. The kidneys maintain the internal milieu so that the rest of the body can thrive. Still, how many people really notice the "Waste Management" truck as it goes about its business once a week?

The kidneys though are more than "Waste Management". The kidneys are important in maintaining our blood pressure, controlling the production of our Red Blood Cells, activating Vitamin D and of course keeping our electrolytes and our acid-base balance in good control.

The kidneys are located immediately in front of the large muscles lateral to the spine. They are in the retroperitoneal space, the space behind the peritoneum, and thus are not really in the abdominal cavity. The kidneys drain into the ureters which empty into the urinary bladder where the urine is stored temporarily. The urethra then drains the bladder. Capping each kidney is an adrenal gland which make cortisone and other hormones.

The kidneys are located at about the level of the second lumbar vertebra. Because of the large liver on the right side which pushes the right kidney down a bit, the left kidney is slightly higher than the right. They are about 5 inches in length and a little less than 3 inches wide and about an inch and a half deep.

When the kidney is sliced along its long axis and filed it is evident that it is divided into three parts: a dark brown colored outer cortex, a lighter-colored medulla and a large fluid-filled hilum which empties into the ureter and through which the kidney's blood vessels pass.

The functional unit of the kidney is the nephron. There are over a million nephrons. The nephron is a long tube which starts in the cortex, drops into the medulla, rises again towards the capsule, only to descend and drain into the hilum. It consists of several parts. The head of the nephron is called Bowman's capsule, inside of which is the glomerulus, a network of capillaries which arise from the renal arteries and ultimately drain into the renal vein. The nephron descends towards the medulla as the proximal convoluted tubule. When it enters the medulla it becomes the Loop of Henle. It then ascends back into the cortex as the distal convoluted tubule which then passes down through the kidney as the collecting duct and drains into the hilum.

The kidneys receive 25% of the cardiac output and twenty percent of the blood passing through the glomerular capillaries is filtered into Bowman's capsule. This represents more than 150 liters of fluid in a day, from which only about 2 liters of urine is produced. Thus the tubules resorb about 148 liters of fluid. This can only occur because the medulla of the kidneys is very high in sodium content, four times greater than serum and because of an active sodium pump energized, of course, by ATP. As the urine passes into the medulla in the descending loop of Henle, water is allowed to pass freely from the dilute urine into the highly concentrated medulla along an osmotic gradient. Most of the water is drained out of the urine.

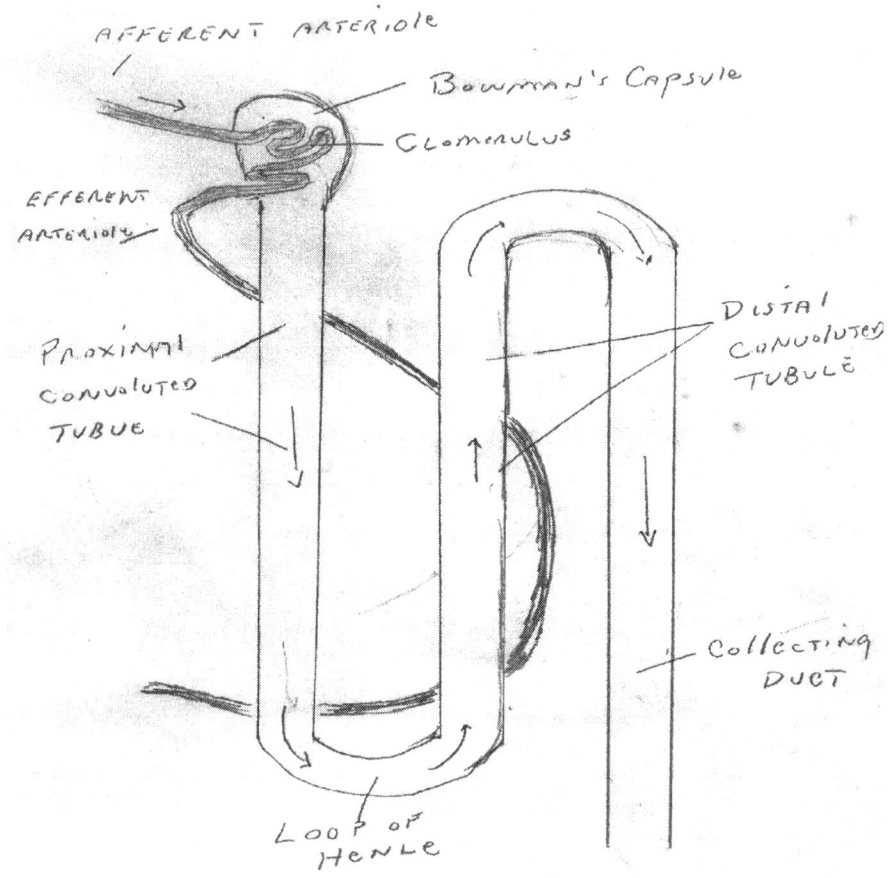

The Nephron

Physiology of the Kidneys

How do the kidneys work? The kidneys have three mechanisms to maintain balance in the body while excreting waste: **filtration, reabsorption and secretion**.

The **filtration** of the blood takes place in Bowman's capsule. The rate of filtration is very high because the lining of the glomerular capillaries is fenestrated (fenestrated comes from the Latin word for window). Water and small molecules pass through without difficulty. Only blood cells and large proteins are unable to pass into the tubular fluid. The filtration of proteins is also inhibited because the basement membrane underlying the endothelial cells has a negative charge and proteins are generally negatively charged. Thus the proteins are repelled by the basement membrane. Like charges repels like just as the south pole on a magnet repels the south pole on a second magnet placed nearby.

The driving force for fluid to leave the glomerulus and enter into the tubule is, in part, due to the difference between the hydrostatic pressure in the glomerulus pushing out and the hydrostatic pressure in Bowman's capsule pushing back against it. The greater the pressure difference the more fluid will be transferred. The other factor involved is the osmotic pressure in the capillary. Since there are no proteins in the tubules only the osmotic pressure in the capillaries matter.

Thus the amount filtered is related to the hydrostatic pressure of the blood (55 mm Hg) minus the sum of the hydrostatic pressure in Bowman's capsule (15 mm Hg) and the osmotic pressure in the blood (30 mm Hg). Thus there is a net filtration pressure of about 10 mm Hg. About 125 cc of fluid/minute are filtered!

Tubular Reabsorption occurs to some extent in the proximal and distal convoluted tubule but more importantly in the Loop of Henle which is the primary site for reabsorption. 99% of water and sodium, 100% of amino acids and sugar, and 50% of urea are reabsorbed. Water absorption is due to osmosis because of the high sodium content of the medulla but sugar is actively absorbed. There is a limit on how much sugar can be reabsorbed. Thus when the blood sugar is greater than 180 mg/100 cc, sugar is lost in the urine.

Reabsorption can be **active**. ATP is used to activate transporter molecules. This occurs in the absorption of glucose, amino acids, minerals and positive ions such as Ca ++, which is under the control of Parathormone (PTH), and Na+, which is partially under the control of Aldosterone. Reabsorption can also be **passive**. When positive ions are absorbed, negative ions are "dragged" with them. The third mechanism is via **osmosis**. Following the absorption of minerals, the filtrate becomes more dilute and water flows along an osmotic gradient into the surrounding capillaries. But the absorption of water is partially under the control of the Antidiuretic Hormone (ADH) in the distal convoluted tubule. ADH is important in that it maintains the blood volume and blood pressure. Lastly reabsorption can be via **pinocytosis** in which the cells lining the tubule engulf chemicals such as small proteins that managed to get through the glomerular endothelium into the tubule.

Lastly **Tubular Secretion** is involved in the control of the hydrogen and potassium ions. Both the ions H+ and K+ are secreted as are the chemicals Ammonia and Creatinine. <u>Most of the H + and K + found in the urine is due to active secretion!</u> Thus active secretion regulates the amount of H+ and K+ in the blood.

The kidneys use these mechanisms to maintain the working environment of the cells of the entire body. The kidneys are the most important part of the body regulating first and foremost the extracellular fluid. They do this by controlling the solutes dissolved in the fluid, including sodium and potassium, which are either retained or lost in the urine.

Water is held in the body in two compartments: the extracellular fluid (ECF) and the intracellular fluid (ICF). The ECF is the total volume of fluid outside the cell. It accounts for one-third of the total body water or about 20% of the total body weight. The ECF includes the plasma, the fluid held within the walls of the blood vessels, and the interstitial fluid, the fluid outside the blood vessels. Note that the blood volume and plasma volume are not the same thing. Forty percent of the blood is red blood cells! <u>The ICF amounts to about two-thirds of the total body water or about 40% of the total body weight.</u> Thus there is twice as much water inside the cells compared to outside the cells. The fluid can pass freely between these compartments and does so based solely on the osmolarity, which is a measure of the concentration of solutes, of the fluid compartments. Because the ECF is in direct contact with the kidneys it is the most easily regulated.

Because sodium is the dominant cation or positively charged ion in the extracellular fluid its excretion is tied directly to total extracellular fluid volume. While every segment of the tubule reabsorbs sodium, the proximal tubule is responsible for two-thirds of the total resorbed sodium. Transport is largely <u>active</u> using the Na-K ATPase cellular channels.

When the pressure in the afferent arteriole is high, meaning the blood pressure is too high or there is too much ECF, tubular resorption will be decreased. Since water follows sodium, more water will be lost and the extracellular fluid volume will decrease. This will lower the blood pressure and decrease the extracellular fluid. The converse is also true.

Hormonal influences play a role as well. When the blood pressure falls, the renin-angiotensin-aldosterone system (RAAS) is activated. In response to low blood pressure, the juxtaglomerular cells of the kidney release renin. The renin converts angiotensinogen, secreted by the liver, into angiotensin 1. An enzyme in the lungs called Angiotensin Converting Enzyme, converts angiotensin 1 to angiotensin 2. Angiotensin 2 is one of the most powerful vasoconstrictors. It directly raises the blood pressure. In addition, the angiotensin 2 stimulates the adrenal glands to release Aldosterone, which acts on the kidneys to make them retain sodium and excrete potassium. Lastly angiotensin 2 causes the hypothalamus to activate the thirst sensation. All these functions will increase the extracellular fluid volume.

Two other hormonal systems are important as well in regulating the ECF. The sympathetic nervous system also stimulates sodium resorption which increases the ECF. Lastly, atrial natriuretic peptide, which is found in the right atrium and which responds to increased volume of the right atrium, reduces sodium resorption and renin secretion. Thus it tends to decrease the ECF.

Potassium (K) regulation is more complicated because most of the potassium is in the ICF and not in the ECF. In fact, only two percent of the body's potassium is in the ECF. Despite this the serum potassium must be tightly regulated. The normal level must be maintained between 3.5 and 5 mEq/L. Too low a potassium level causes profound weakness while too high a potassium level will cause serious cardiac arrhythmias and even death. Because precise control of the potassium level is needed, two mechanisms are involved. The first and fastest, taking only seconds, is the movement of potassium directly between the ECF and ICF. This is accomplished using an active cellular transport channel that exchanges the potassium ion for the hydrogen ion. For example when we eat a typical meal we ingest about to 40 mEq of potassium even though the total ECF pool is only 60 mEq. The potassium absorbed from our food must be shifted rapidly from the ECF to the ICF to avoid a fatal spike in our serum potassium level. This reaction is amplified by insulin which increases the Na-K ATPase. Beta adrenergic agents and the hormone aldosterone have a similar effect.

When we exercise strenuously ICF potassium flows into the ECF raising the serum level. When we develop an acidosis, the hydrogen ions flow into the cells in exchange for potassium again raising the serum level. To prevent serious consequences from exercise or acidosis, a second mechanism must be called into play. Renal tubular potassium absorption and excretion is responsible for the long-term control of total body potassium stores. Nearly two-thirds of the filtered potassium is resorbed in the proximal tubule while another quarter of the tubular potassium is resorbed in the ascending loop of Henle by a NA-2Cl-K active transport system. Fine regulation of the potassium however occurs near the end of the distal tubule and in the collecting ducts. When extracellular potassium is low, cells of this part of the nephron resorb nearly all of the intra-tubular potassium in exchange for the hydrogen ion, probably using the H-K ATPase channels. When ECF potassium is high, certain cells of the distal convoluted tubule and collecting ducts excrete potassium into the tubule, again in exchange for hydrogen ions, using a NA-K ATPase channel.

Respiratory therapists need to be aware of these relationships. For example, when they give a treatment to a patient using Albuterol they are using a Beta adrenergic agent which will facilitate the transfer of potassium from the ECF to the ICF. If the patient already has low potassium, a further drop in the ion could cause a fatal cardiac arrhythmia! Therefore, The RT's should check the laboratory results to see what the patient's potassium is before treating the patient!

Another example: anything which causes low potassium will cause a metabolic alkalosis as the kidney retains potassium by secreting hydrogen in exchange (the K-H ATPase channel exchanges K for K). So a patient who is on a diuretic which causes a depletion of potassium will develop a metabolic alkalosis. The key to good patient care is to review the patient's history, listen to the patient's lung sounds, check his or her laboratory findings and review the list of the medications the patient is receiving.

The kidneys are important in regulating acid-base balance. They help maintain acid-base balance through their ability to regulate tubular secretion of H^+ and reabsorption of HCO_3. The renal tubules are capable of secreting H^+ when blood pH is acidic. The rate of secretion is directly proportional to H^+ concentration in blood and thus there is an increase in secretion when the blood is more acidic. The renal tubules can also excrete HCO_3 ion into the urine when blood pH is alkaline.

Diseases of the Kidneys

The kidneys can fail in two ways. If the glomerulus becomes too leaky and allows large proteins to escape from the blood into the tubule the protein level in the blood will fall dramatically. The patient will become weak. In addition, since the proteins in the blood are responsible for holding water inside the capillaries because of their effect on osmotic pressure, water will escape the blood into the interstitial space resulting in generalized edema. This condition is called the *nephrotic syndrome*. The renal function, as measured by the blood urea nitrogen or creatinine level, may often be normal because the renal tubules are still functioning. The nephrotic syndrome is often caused by an autoimmune disease such as systemic lupus erythematosus. The nephrotic syndrome is also associated with clots forming in the renal veins and causing pulmonary emboli.

More commonly renal failure is caused by failure of the nephrons to secrete or absorb chemicals and waste materials. Renal failure is detected by a **decrease or absence of urine production** or by an **increase of waste products such as creatinine or urea in the blood**. Depending on the cause, hematuria, blood in the urine and proteinuria, which is protein in the urine, may also be noted.

There are three types of renal failure: prerenal, renal, or obstructive.

If the blood pressure falls in the glomerulus, the *glomerular filtration rate* or the rate at which blood is filtered in the glomerulus will fall. The decrease in the fluid sent down into the rest of the tubule will affect how much of the solutes are resorbed. This is called *prerenal failure* and is seen in patients with congestive heart failure or shock. If the onset is acute, the patient may present with oliguria or decreased urine volumes.

A second cause of renal failure is disease of the kidney itself. The main parts of the tubule become diseased. This can be either acute or chronic. In acute renal failure, there is rapidly progressive loss of renal function, generally characterized by oliguria, which means decreased urine production to less than 400 mL per day in adults, as well as fluid and electrolyte imbalances. This is often caused by acute ischemia to the kidney due to tissue hypoxia or by certain forms of glomerular disease in which the glomeruli become scarred rather than "leaky". Chronic disease develops gradually and most often is due to diabetes, long-standing infection or inflammation of the nephrons called pyelonephritis, chronic gout or a metabolic condition such as hypocalcemia. Other causes include tubular diseases such as tubular necrosis or obstruction of the renal tubules by uric acid crystals. Waste products, such as urea, build up in the blood and electrolyte imbalances occur.

Lastly, renal failure can be due to blockage of the outflow of the kidneys causing a back pressure referred to as obstructive uropathy.

Symptoms of renal failure are protean. High levels of urea cause nausea and vomiting resulting in dehydration and weight loss. Increased phosphates cause itching, muscle cramps (due to low calcium from the increased phosphate ion) and metabolic acidosis. This may also occur because kidneys are unable to conserve the bicarbonate ion. Increased potassium levels causes cardiac arrhythmias and muscle weakness. Finally, increased water retention causes peripheral edema and shortness of breath due to pulmonary edema.

The treatment of renal failure depends totally upon identifying the cause and fixing the underlying disorder, if possible. If a cause can't be found or if the disease progresses then dialysis or renal transplantation are the only options.

Other Functions of the Kidney

The kidneys are important in blood pressure regulation. The juxtaglomerular cells, the cells next to the glomerulus, secrete renin which activates angiotensin and raises the blood pressure.

The kidneys also secrete erythropoietin. When the patient becomes hypoxic, erythropoietin is secreted by the kidneys which stimulates the bone marrow to make more red blood cells. When the kidneys fail, they produce less erythropoietin resulting in decreased production of red blood cells and anemia. The patient develops weakness and fatigue. Dialysis does not correct the anemia but a kidney transplant will.

Lastly, the kidneys are important in the activation of Vitamin D. Vitamin D increases the absorption of Calcium and Phosphate from the gut. Without vitamin D, the patient will develop osteomalacia or weak bones.

Lecture Notes: Anatomy and Physiology for the Respiratory Therapist

Part Two: Acid-Base Balance

The kidneys are especially important to the respiratory therapist because they are responsible for one-half of the body's acid-base regulation. The other half, of course, is the lungs. In order to gain an understanding of acid-base balance we need to know what acids and bases are. An **acid** is a chemical which can **donate** a hydrogen + ion (proton):

$$H Cl \text{ (hydrochloric acid)} > H+ \; + \; Cl-$$

$$H_2CO_3 \text{ (carbonic acid)} > H+ \; + \; HCO_3-$$

$$HC_2H_3O_2 \text{ (acetic acid)} > H+ \; + \; C_2H_3O_2-$$

Acids can be "strong" or "weak" depending upon how easily they "dissociate" or, in other words, give up their H+ ion. Strong acids like HCl give up their H+ easily. Weak acids like H_2CO_3 give up their H+ with difficulty. Strong acids such as HCl or hydrochloric acid, "dissociate" completely. They release all their H+ ions or protons. Weak acids such as H_2CO_3 or carbonic acid, "dissociate" only partially. For hydrochloric acid, the concentration of H+ is extremely high at about 10^{-2}.

A **base**, on the other hand, **accepts** a hydrogen ion

$$NaOH \text{ (sodium hydroxide)} + H+ \; > HOH + Na+$$

The NaOH forms a Na+ and an OH-. The OH- then takes up the free H+ in the solution to form water. Other examples of a base include:

$$NH_3 \text{ (ammonia)} + H+ \; > NH_4+ \text{ (the ammonium ion)}$$

$$HCO_3- \text{ (bicarbonate ion)} + H+ \; > H_2CO_3$$

How do we measure the acidity of the blood? The scale we use is the pH scale. *The pH is the negative **log** of the hydrogen ion in the solution.* Water has 10^{-7} moles of hydrogen ions per liter. The negative log of 10^{-7} is 7. Because water has an equal amount of hydrogen and hydroxyl ions it is "neutral". That means that the number of H+ ions equals the number of OH- ions. A pH of less than 7 means there is an excess of H+, while a pH of more than 7 means there is an excess of hydrogen ion receptors such as OH-. Most importantly a **unit** change in the pH represents a tenfold change in the hydrogen concentration. Thus if the pH of a solution goes from 7 to 6 there is ten times more hydrogen ion in solution. It is only the free H+ that determines the pH (the concentration of the H+ ion). In other words, the acidity is directly related to the proton or hydrogen ion concentration.

The pH of common solutions varies widely. Bleach has a pH of 12, while milk of magnesia has a pH of 10.5. Saltwater is more "basic" than tap water with a pH of 8.4 compared to tap water's 7. Coffee is acidic with a pH of 5, tomato juice has a pH of 4.2 and lemon juice is very acidic with a pH of 2.

What is the pH of our blood? The pH of our blood is tightly controlled with a range between 7.35 and 7.45. The maintenance of the acid-base homeostasis is accomplished by: 1. the buffer systems of the body which are the first line of defense and act immediately; 2. the rate and depth of respiration which acts within a few minutes; and 3. the kidneys, which while the most effective system, take a couple of days to work.

What is a *buffer*? A buffer is the salt of a weak acid. NaHCO3 (sodium bicarbonate) is the salt of H2CO3 (carbonic acid). A buffer ameliorates ("buffers") the reaction. Thus when HCl, a very strong acid, is added to a solution containing NaHCO3, you end up with H2CO3, a very weak acid, and NaCl or table salt.

HCl + <u>NaHCO3</u> > H2CO3 + NaCl

HCl is hydrochloric acid which is quite a strong acid

NaHCO3 is the salt of the weak acid

H2CO3 is carbonic acid which is a weak acid.

Buffers are important to prevent sudden, large changes in the acidity or alkalinity of the blood and tissues. There are three buffer systems in our blood: 1. NaHCO3, which is the salt of H2CO3, 2. NaH2PO4 (sodium mono-hydrogen-phosphate) which is the salt of NaH2PO4, and 3. Hemoglobin and other circulating proteins. **Hemoglobin and proteins are the major buffer system in the intracellular fluid.** Proteins are made up of amino acids which contain a carboxyl and an amino group. The carboxyl group (COOH) acts as a weak acid and the amino group (NH2) acts as a weak base.

The carbonic acid system is the most important buffer because it is controlled by both the lungs and the kidneys. When CO2 is combined with water the result is H2CO3 or carbonic acid which then breaks down into H+ and HCO3-. The lungs can directly raise or lower the CO2 while the kidneys can raise or lower the HCO3-.

Why is the system so important? The kidney regulates the HCO3- via the tubular reabsorption of HCO3- and secretion of H+ ion. The kidneys secrete H + ion into the renal filtrate and return HCO3 - to the blood. Either CO2 or NH3 can be used to secrete H+. If CO2 is used it combines with water or H2O to give H2CO3 which breaks down into H+ and HCO3-. The HCO3 is absorbed back into the blood while the H+ passes into the nephron and out the urine. NH3 or ammonia can combine with H + to give NH4+ which is secreted into the filtrate as NH4CL (ammonium chloride) thus eliminating the H+. For each H + secreted into the filtrate a Na+ must be reabsorbed. The main problem the renal system is that it takes 24 to 36 hours to react. *Importantly, only the renal system can regulate alkaline substances in the blood.*

The lungs regulate the CO2 (H2CO3). The reaction occurs nearly instantly though it is still not as fast as the chemical buffers. **Nevertheless the pulmonary system has twice the buffering capacity of all the chemical buffers in the blood combined!** Normally, the amount of CO2 excreted in the lungs is equal to the amount of CO2 produced by the tissues, but the lung can adjust the amount of CO2 excreted by changes in the rate and depth of respiration.

The Henderson-Hasselbach equation shows the relationship between the pH, the HCO3- and H2CO3. When any two variables of the equation are known, the third can always be calculated.

pH = Pka + log (HCO3-/H2CO3)

Where H2CO3 equals 0.03 X pCO2 and the pKa is 6.1

For example, if a patient has a HCO3- of 24 and a pCO2 of 40, we can calculate the pH.

1. From the equation (H2CO3 = 0.03 X pCO2) we get a H2CO3 of 1.2.
2. Then, from the equation (pH = Pka + log (HCO3-/H2CO3)) we calculate that the pH = 6.1 + log 24/1.2.
3. Solving the equation gives us a pH = 6.1 + log of 20 which is 6.1 + 1.3 or 7.4.

If the pCO2 doubles to 80, the H2CO2 will be 2.4 and the equation becomes (pH = 6.1 + log of 24/2.4) or (6.1 + 1) which is 7.1. Thus doubling the CO2 decreases the pH by 0.3.

Diseases which affect the HCO3- directly are **metabolic disorders**. A **metabolic acidosis** is an acidosis associated with a decreased HCO3. Common causes include:

1. lactic acidosis due to "shock"
2. diabetic ketoacidosis due to the build-up of ketones
3. renal failure due to the accumulation of phosphates and sulfates
4. the ingestion of aspirin, after all aspirin is acetyl salicylic acid
5. the ingestion of alcohol
6. ingestion of ethylene glycol

All of these conditions are characterized as having an increased **anion gap.**

Anion Gap = Na+ - (Cl- + HCO3-)

Normal = < 14

On the other hand a **metabolic alkalosis** is an alkalotic condition associated with an increased HCO3. Some of the causes of metabolic alkalosis include:

1. hypokalemia in which the kidneys conserve K+ by excreting H+
2. hypochloremia or low Cl- which causes the kidneys to conserve HCO3- in order to maintain the balance between anions and cations
3. vomiting or gastric suctioning which causes the loss of Cl-
4. steroids such as prednisone which cause the kidneys to excrete K+ and H+ ions
5. diuretics which cause the renal excretion of Cl- and H+
6. administration of excessive HCO3-
7. hypovolemia which causes the excretion of H +

Diseases which affect the carbon dioxide directly are called respiratory disorders. **Respiratory Acidosis** associated with a high CO2. This can be due to:

1. COPD

2. central nervous system depression due to drug overdose or anesthesia
3. neurologic disorders including Guillain-Barre and myasthenia gravis

Respiratory Alkalosis is characterized by a low CO2 and can be due to:

1. CNS disorders such as meningitis which causes hyperventilation
2. hypoxemia
3. emotional disorder such as pain or anxiety)
4. The third trimester of pregnancy.

Given time, some compensation will occur to ameliorate the acute acid-base disorder. If the patient develops a metabolic acidosis due to shock, he will have a sudden drop in his pH, but the lungs will partially compensate through hyperventilation. This will "blow off" CO2 and partially normalize the pH. On the other hand if a patient has chronic bronchitis and an increased CO2 due to "hypoventilation", the kidneys will retain HCO3- in order to bring the pH back to normal.

The ability of the lungs and kidneys to compensate for acute changes makes interpreting blood gases and acid-base balance a little more difficult.

How do I interpret the acid base status from a blood gas? For me, the first step is to check the pH. Is it acidic or basic? Is the pH less than 7.4 or more than 7.4? Then I look at the pCO2. Does it agree with the change in pH? If the pH is low while the CO2 is high, then we must have a respiratory acidosis. If the pH is low but the CO2 is normal or low then we must have a metabolic acidosis. Lastly, I look at the HCO3 to see if it is in the normal range.

If we have a primary respiratory dysfunction, and the HCO3 is normal, then we have an uncompensated condition. If it isn't, then there must be some compensation.

For example, if the blood gases show:

$$pH = 7.2, \ pCO2 = 80, \ HCO3 = 26$$

The pH is low meaning there is an acidosis. The CO2 is high, confirming that this is a respiratory acidosis. The HCO3 is also high suggesting that there has been some renal compensation. Thus, I conclude we have a partially compensated respiratory acidosis. Since the kidneys take days to compensate, this must be at least in part, a chronic respiratory acidosis.

Let's look at one more case:

$$pH = 7.2, \ pCO2 = 24, \ HCO3 = 12$$

The pH is again low, but the CO2 is also low. It can't be a respiratory acidosis. It must be a metabolic acidosis. When we look at the HCO3 we find it is, in fact, quite low. Thus we have a metabolic acidosis. When we look back at the CO2 we realize that it is low because the patient is hyperventilating to compensate for the metabolic acidosis.

We use the blood gases every day to evaluate our patients. It is paramount to clearly understand how the lungs and kidneys work together to maintain the bodies acid-base status.

IMPORTANT CONCEPTS TO REMEMBER FROM THIS LECTURE

1. The functional unit of the kidney is the:

    Nephron

1. The glomerulus is lined by:

    A leaky or fenestrated endothelial lining and negatively charged basement membrane

2. Which ions are actively secreted into the tubular fluid?

    H+ and K+

3. Kidneys aid in maintaining normal acid-base balance through:

    The absorption and secretion of HCO3- and the secretion of H+

4. Low potassium can cause a:

    Metabolic alkalosis

Peter A. Petroff, MD

Lecture Twenty

Fetal Development and Aging

Where do the lungs come from? How fast do the lungs grow? What kind of tissue gives rise to lung tissue?

When a sperm successfully fertilizes an egg, the egg will burrow into the wall of the uterus. The site where this occurs becomes the placenta which will provide oxygen and nutrients to the developing fetus and carry waste products and carbon dioxide away from the fetus. The fetus grows explosively. A primitive heart structure, gut, and nervous system form rapidly.

The lung develops in stages. The first stage of lung development is the "budding" of tissue from the esophagus. About the 24th day after conception a small mass of tissue buds from the anterior esophagus. Within a few days the bud has divided in two tiny masses of tissue. After another eleven days, cartilage can be found in the bud and by day forty-two all the lung segments are present though quite undeveloped. Following this is the "pseudoglandular" phase which occurs over the next four weeks. Cartilage, smooth muscle and immature glands appear.

The period of time from the 17th to 24th weeks after conception is the "Canalicular" period. Terminal bronchioles proliferate and a few respiratory bronchioles appear. Vascularization of the lungs begins and distinct lobes are present. Even lymphatics begin to make their appearance.

From week 24 to birth is the "terminal sac period". The alveoli develop and Type 1 and 2 alveolar cells are found as is Surfactant. The smooth muscles fibers mature. <u>By the 28th week the air-blood interface and the amount of Surfactant present is enough to support life.</u>

There are three types of tissue in the fetus: the ectoderm or outer layer which will become the skin and its contiguous tissues as well as the eyes, ear and nervous system, the endoderm or inner layer which forms the gut and the lungs and finally the mesoderm or middle layer which forms the muscles, bones, the underlying layers of the skin (dermis), kidneys, heart and most blood vessels.

Thus with the exception of one cell type, the airways and alveoli develop from the *endoderm*, the tissue lining the gut. Moreover, the lung and the gut are exquisitely intertwined from the time of conception. That relationship will last throughout the person's life.

The one type of cell not from the endoderm comes instead from the primitive spinal cord, called the *"neural crest."* These cells are the pigment stained, neuroendocrine cells, the K cells or Kulchinsky cells. They are also called Enterochromaffin cells.

The trachea, bronchi, bronchioles and alveoli are thus derived from endoderm. By the fifth month there are already 17 generations of branching of bronchi and bronchioles. By the 7th month alveolar ducts are present and by the 8th month alveoli are well developed. The bronchial tubes invade the mesoderm, which then forms part of the supporting structure such as cartilage, muscle, and fibrous tissue including the visceral pleura.

The placenta forms at the site of implantation of the fertilized egg. It is a complex structure. Maternal blood flows into small vessels called the spiral arterioles which drain into the intervillous space. The intervillous space surrounds the chorionic villa in which the fetal capillaries from the fetal umbilical artery are present. These capillaries merge to form the umbilical veins which go from the placenta to the fetus.

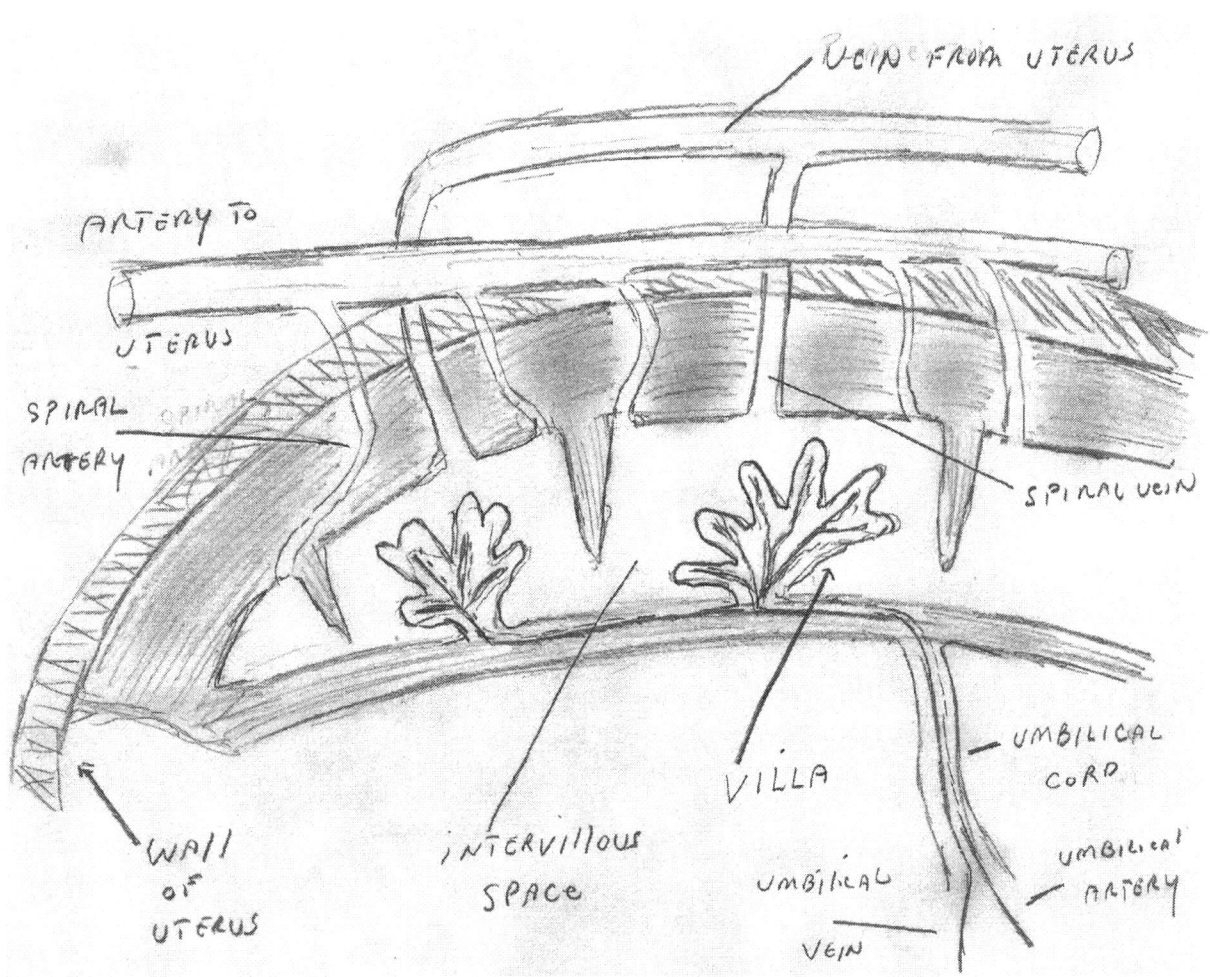

The Placenta

Maternal blood flows from the uterine arteries to the placenta where small spiral branches enter the intervillous space. Blood returns to the uterus via spiral veins. On the fetal side, blood from the umbilical artery in the umbilical cord enters the villas where they are oxygenated. The blood then leaves via the umbilical vein.

It is difficult to imagine but the fetal paO2 is only about 30 and the paCO2 is 40. The fetus is able to survive with these blood gases because the fetus has a different form of hemoglobin (Hemoglobin F instead of hemoglobin A as in the adult) which takes up the O2 more efficiently. In addition, the fetus has more hemoglobin to start with.

To understand the fetal circulation we must remember that blood flowing towards the heart is a vein and blood flowing away from the heart is an artery. The fetal blood flowing from the placenta towards the fetus is the umbilical vein, not artery because it flows towards the heart. The blood flowing from the fetus to the placenta is the umbilical artery, even though it has much less oxygen than the umbilical vein!

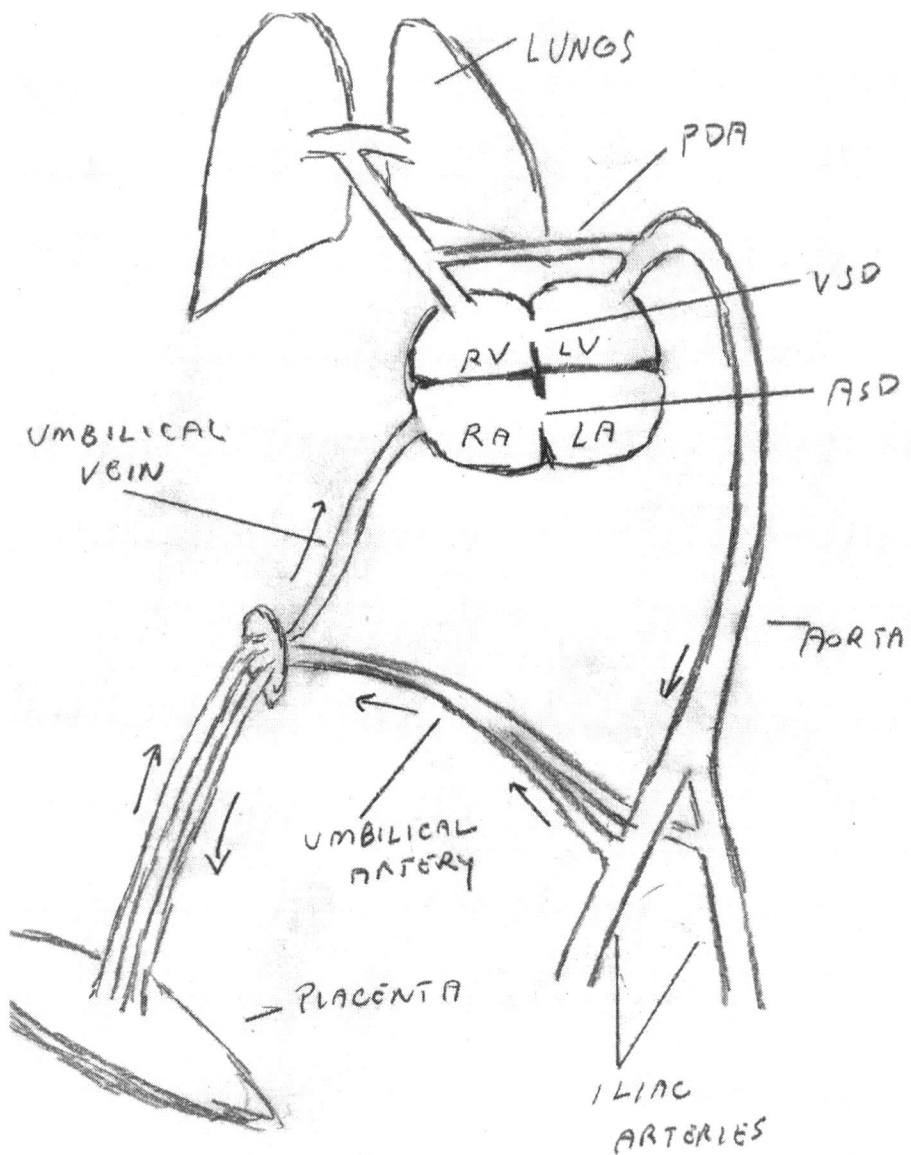

Fetal Circulation

Blood flows from the placenta to the fetus via the umbilical vein. The PaO2 is about 30 with a paCO2 of about 40. Half of the blood goes to the liver (Ductus Venosus) and half enters the inferior vena cava. From there the blood enters the right atrium and then most of the blood flows directly into the left atrium via a patent Foramen Ovale. The blood in the left atrium enters the left ventricle then the aorta. Some of the blood flows out the pulmonary artery but is quickly shunted into the aorta by the ductus arteriosus. **<u>Before birth, only 15% of the blood actually reaches the lung tissue.</u>**

The aorta gives rise to common Iliac Arteries which branch into External and Internal Iliac Arteries. The Umbilical Artery is a branch of the Internal Iliac Artery. In the Umbilical Artery the paO2 is about 20 and the paCO2 is about 55. Blood flows from the umbilical artery to the placenta to become oxygenated, to pick up nutrients, and to eliminate carbon dioxide and waste products.

In the fetus, the oxygenated blood is carried in the Umbilical Vein and the deoxygenated blood in the Umbilical Artery.

Birth is a momentous occasion, to say the least. After birth the placenta is expelled, the umbilical arteries atrophy, the umbilical vein becomes the Round Ligament of the liver, The Ductus Venosus becomes the fibrous cord of the liver, the Foramen Ovale closes and finally the Ductus Arteriosus atrophies and becomes the Ligamentum Arteriosum.

Why does the baby take its first breath? The peripheral and central receptors are inactive during fetal life but at birth become active and are probably responsible for initiating the first breath.

When the infant is driven to inhale for the first time, which requires a negative pleural pressure of about -100 cm H20, air fills the alveoli. With the rise in the alveolar oxygen level, the pulmonary resistance falls dramatically and most of the blood entering the right atrium now flows out into the lungs. The pressure in the left atrium rises and shuts the Foramen Ovale. Complete closure in most people occurs at about 9 months, but patent Foramen Ovale (Atrial Septal Defects) have been found in patients presenting with congestive heart failure in their 60's.

The increased paO2 results in closure of the ductus arteriosus which eventually becomes a fibrous cord. In a few infants, the ductus fails to close and the infant develops pulmonary hypertension.

What do the pulmonary function studies look like in a newborn infant? The newborn's tidal volume is about 15 ml, Total Lung Capacity is about 155 ml, and the Vital Capacity is about 115 ml. The baby breathes about 40 times a minute and has a heart rate of about 140. His or her blood pressure is about 65/40. At birth the blood gases show a pH of about 7.2, pCO2 of about 55 and a pO2 of about 55. Within 72 hours, the blood gases become normal.

Doctors evaluate how a newborn is doing by using the Apgar Score. It consists of five factors: heart rate, respiratory effort, muscle tone, reflex irritability and color. Each factor gets a score of 0 to 2. The baby is considered out of danger when the score is greater than 7.

The Respiratory Therapist needs to be aware of three reflexes that are truly very important in the newborn. The first is the Trigeminal Reflex. Stimulation of the face, nose and nasopharyngeal mucosa causes a decrease in respiration and heart rate. The therapist must exercise extreme care in suctioning the newborn. The second reflux is the Irritant Reflex. In the preterm infant, irritation of the mucosa of the airway causes a slowing of respiration while in the full term it causes hyperventilation. Lastly, Head's Paradoxical Reflex is extremely important. When the newborn takes a breath, it often will take a further deep inspiration. This is similar to a sigh and may be important in preventing alveolar collapse. The opposite reflex, the Herring Breuer reflex, which is found in adults, whereby a deep breath causes cessation of inhalation, is inactive in newborns.

What can go wrong? The most common problem is the Respiratory Distress Syndrome (Hyaline Membrane Disease) which affect 50% of infants born about the 28th week of gestation and 25% born in the 30th week of gestation It occurs because of inadequate amounts of Surfactant, which results in increased surface tension in the alveoli causing atelectasis. Pathologic findings include: hyaline membrane formation, areas of pulmonary hemorrhage, atelectasis, interstitial and alveolar edema. These abnormalities result in severe hypoxemia. Clinically, the infant is tachypneic with nasal flaring, intercostal retractions and grunting. On examination there are bilateral inspiratory crackles. The chest x-ray shows a ground glass appearance. The treatment is the inhalation of Surfactant as well as positive pressure breathing.

After birth, the lungs continue to develop. At birth there are 17 generations of branching but by adult age there are 24. The number of alveoli increases. **At birth there are only 24 million alveoli. By age 12, there are ten times as many, the same number as in adults.** The elastic supporting tissue increases up to age 18. Finally, the thorax changes in shape from cuboidal to rectangular.

Sadly these positive changes do not go on forever! The growth of the lungs is complete by age 20 and the pulmonary function studies reach their maximum between age 20 and 25. From there on out, lung function, like the rest of our physiology, steadily and ruthlessly wanes!

When we are a child we look forward to growing. Shortly after his fifth birthday the young man will say, "I'm almost six!" But by the time she is thirty and a day before her thirty-first birthday she will still say, "I'm only thirty." We all fear aging, I suppose, and with good reason. No part of our body is unaffected by growing older. Every organ is affected, from our brain to our kidneys and that, of course, includes the lungs.

The elderly are those people over 60. They are making up a larger and larger share of the world's population. In countries like Japan, Germany and the United States they will soon be in the majority as population growth in those there countries has fallen below sustainability levels.

What can we expect as we age? Sadly with advancing age the capacity of the brain steadily declines. Even the brain size falls after the age of 45. Cognition (thinking and understanding) becomes more of a problem even in normal people. Some degree of memory loss becomes apparent. Blood flow to the brain decreases. All this results in a decreased ability to solve unfamiliar complex problems. Cerebellar function (the back part of the brain responsible for balance and coordinating movement) declines fastest of all, resulting in an increased risk of falling.

Cardiac function decreases about 1% a year after the age of 30. The cardiac output of a man of 80 is half that of a twenty-year old. As we age, the cardiac muscle becomes less responsive to catecholamines, the muscle becomes stiffer likely due to interstitial fibrosis of the myocardial tissue, amyloid (proteinaceous) deposits are found in the heart muscle, especially the atria, which leads to heart arrhythmias and contribute to the stiffness of the myocardium; the afterload increases because of increased blood pressure due to atherosclerotic blood vessels and increased vascular resistance.

Muscle mass also decreases with aging. While the diaphragm is spared from the aging process, the other muscles of respiration are not. Fat replaces muscle! In addition osteoarthritis and degenerative joint disease stiffen the spine and chest wall making the chest wall stiffer (less compliant).

The lungs become more emphysematous, even in never-smokers. The number of alveoli decrease and the elastic supporting structure of the lung deteriorates. This results in decreased elastic recoil and the tendency of the small airways to collapse during exhalation. This change is seen mainly at the base of the lung, causing increased ventilation/perfusion inequality.

The kidneys are affected as well. A 90 year old man has 30% less kidney function than he had when he was thirty. By age 65, the number of glomeruli have decreased from 1 million to seven hundred thousand. Tubular function is impaired as well which results in the elderly being more susceptible to dehydration and hyponatremia.

Even the gastrointestinal tract is not spared from the effects of growing old. Movement of a bolus of food is slowed passing through the esophagus because of decreased peristalsis and decreased ability to open the lower esophageal sphincter. These changes will, of course, increase the risk of aspiration. At the other end of the GI tract, constipation becomes a constant problem and stool incontinence occurs all too frequently.

The main factors affecting the lung are the generalized weakness in muscle tissue, the increased stiffness of the thorax, the decreased cardiac function, and, of course, the decreased alveoli and loss of the elastic supporting structure of the lung resulting in small airways dysfunction.

Because of these changes the Vital Capacity decreases 20-25 ml/year and the FEV1 decreases 20-30 ml/year. Only the total lung capacity does NOT change with aging. The increase pulmonary compliance is balanced by the muscle weakness. Nevertheless the muscle loss, combined with early small airway closure, causes the RV and RV/TLC ratio to increase. At age 30 the RV/TLC ratio is about 20; at age sixty it is 35!

In addition, as the chest wall becomes stiffer there is a decrease in chest wall compliance resulting in a higher FRC. (Note that the ERV actually decreases a little.) **Thus the FRC and the RV both increase. The vital capacity falls as the RV increases though the TLC remains unchanged.** The VC decreases 25 ml a year so that by age 70 it has decreased about 40-50%.

The muscle weakness causes reduced forced expiration. The FVC decreases about 22 cc/yr in men and 20 cc/yr in women. The loss of alveoli results in decreased diffusion. It falls about 25% over the life of an individual. Finally, the loss of alveoli combined with the small airways disease leads to an increase in dead space ventilation with age.

The $pAO_2 - paO_2$ gradient increases as well. The paO_2 falls from about 90 to 75 however, the $paCO_2$ remains normal. The P(A-a) O_2 difference increases with aging, likely related to changes in the physiologic dead space.

Two significant other changes seen in the elderly include: 1. the older patient becomes less responsiveness to hypoxia and hypercapnia, and 2. mucociliary transport is reduced as well perhaps due to dehydration thickening the double-layered mucous gel.

Summary of pulmonary changes:

FACTOR	In the elderly
Total lung capacity	normal
Vital capacity	decreased by half
Functional residual capacity	increases
Residual lung volume	increases
RV/TLC ratio	nearly doubled
Diffusion	decreases
Ventilation/perfusion ratio	increases
pAO2 – paO2 gradient	increases

But Exercise ability is impaired <u>because of the fall in cardiac output</u> not the changes in the lungs! The heart becomes stiff due to fibrosis.

<u>The maximum heart rate decreases steadily with aging</u>. The Maximum heart rate is 220 minus the age. At twenty it is 200. At 70 it is 150.

Stroke volume and Cardiac Output decrease. Peripheral vascular resistance increases. Aerobic capacity falls by 50%.

With advancing age the blood pressure increases, stroke volume decreases and heart work decreases.

Can we prevent these changes? Exercise is the answer. Exercise decreases the BP, decreases cardiac muscle stiffness, increases bone density, increases muscle mass and strength, decreases body fat and blood sugar, Decreases LDL (the bad cholesterol), raises HDL (the good cholesterol), improves sleep and improves memory.

IMPORTANT CONCEPTS TO REMEMBER FROM THIS LECTURE

1. The K cell or Kulchinsky cell is the precursor of small cell cancer. It develops from what kind of tissue?

    Primitive neural crest

2. The PaO2 in the umbilical artery (the artery to the fetus) is about?

    30

3. The number of alveoli reach their adult value by the age of?

    Twelve

4. Pulmonary function values reaches their maximum by the age of?

    Twenty to twenty five

5. With aging, exercise ability is decreased because of a fall in the FEV1?

    False

Peter A. Petroff, MD

Lecture Twenty-one

Exercise, Diving and Exposure to High Altitude

Humankind has always been a curious lot, never satisfied with the status quo. But unlike other creatures who never seem to learn from their curiosity, and suffer the consequences, humankind studies and learns from their explorations, whether it be climbing the highest mountain, exploring the depths of the sea or even voyaging to other worlds.

Our world is miraculous in that it can support so many kinds of life so very well. Bacteria have even been found living in the middle of rocks with no access to water or oxygen! But living at high altitudes, diving underwater, or even exercising at the gym can stress our ability to cope. While the fraction of oxygen is constant from the top of Mount Everest to the bottom of Death Valley, the partial pressure of oxygen varies with atmospheric pressure. At the top of Mount Everest the barometric pressure is 253 torr so that the atmospheric oxygen is 53 torr. In a study done in 1983 by J. B. West and his associates, the alveolar oxygen of healthy young climbers was only 35 torr! The alveolar carbon dioxide was 7.5 torr. The arterial pH was 7.7! A recent British study showed that the amount of hemoglobin concentration increased at higher altitudes during acclimation. Even though the amount of oxygen in the air fell as did the arterial oxygen saturation, the total amount of oxygen in the blood fell much less due to the increased hemoglobin and a shift to the left of the hemoglobin saturation curve.

Diving to great depths presents its own problems. With increased pressure the chest wall is squeezed and the lung volumes fall dramatically. In addition there is a shift in nitrogen from the blood into the tissues which can create problems when the diver surfaces. The bubbles of nitrogen in the tissues expand and cause the "bends" which are often fatal.

Even exercising has its problems. During strenuous exercise, oxygen consumption and heat production may increase up to 20 fold and blood flow to the muscles and skin up to 25 fold. The heart and lungs have to compensate dramatically for these changes.

But more and more people are attempting these dangerous challenges. So far this year (as of June, 2019) eleven mountaineers have died climbing Everest! The Nepalese Director of Tourism is concerned that there is "overcrowding" on the most commonly used climbing route to the summit. Two of the most recent deaths were in men over sixty (61 and 64). Twenty years ago no one over sixty would even think about attempting the climb. Interestingly, both men made it to the top. One died a few hours after reaching the top. The other died a day after his ascension.

Diving is also a risk. In 2008, there were 7 million active divers world-wide and more than a half-million are training to be divers every year. There are an average of 100 deaths due to diving and more than a thousand cases of decompression illness every year in the United States alone. While many dive for entertainment, diving is important for offshore oilfield exploration, seafood harvesting, construction, and even anthropology.

Altitude

At sea level, the atmospheric pressure is 760 mm Hg and the inspired O_2 is 159 mm Hg (760 X .21). At a ski resort in Colorado (8,840 feet altitude), the atmospheric pressure is 526 mg Hg, and the inspired O2 is 110 mm Hg. At the top of Mount Everest the atmospheric pressure is 253 and the inspired O2 is 53 mg Hg. When water pressure is subtracted from 253, the alveolar pAO2 is even less (253- 47 = 206; 206 X .21 = 43 mg Hg). Most of the climbers of Mount Everest in the past were professional climbers who took the time to acclimatize to the high attitude thus increasing their blood oxygen but holiday skiers normally live at low altitudes and come up to altitude for a week of fun without any attempt at acclimatization.

How do we adapt to high altitude? The peripheral chemoreceptors, sensitive to decreasing paO2, signal the respiratory centers to increase ventilation. However, because the vital capacity falls in the non-acclimatized skier, the respiratory rate must increase. The fall in vital capacity is likely due to mild interstitial edema. In addition, there is a mild respiratory alkalosis as the paCO2 drops due to the increased alveolar ventilation. The respiratory alkalosis then causes the oxygen hemoglobin saturation curve to shift to the left thus allowing the blood to take up more oxygen as it passes through the lungs. Over 48 hours, some renal compensation occurs decreasing this effect.

Initially, diffusion decreases. With the fall in pAO2 the driving pressure for diffusion, the difference between the alveolar and arterial oxygen concentration, will be reduced and the transit time for blood in the capillaries of the lung may be inadequate for full diffusion to occur. Exercise (skiing) will make this worse due to the increased cardiac output which decreases the transit time still further.

Acclimatization occurs over time. The peripheral chemoreceptors do NOT acclimatize to the low paO2 so that there will always be a degree of alveolar hyperventilation. However, over time the vital capacity increases as do the red blood cells. The hemoglobin concentration can increase up to a hemoglobin concentration of 20.5 at six weeks. Recall, the normal hemoglobin concentration is about 16. The O2 diffusing capacity increases and may be 25% more than lowlanders. This may be due to the improvement in the vital capacity which increases the surface area (A) in the diffusion equation. All these changes result in an improvement in the paO2 over time. Lastly, the myoglobin increases as well, especially in the diaphragm and heart. This improves the transfer of oxygen from the blood to the muscle tissue. It also provides storage for oxygen in the peripheral tissues.

There are several disorders associated with high altitude. **Acute mountain sickness** (AMS) has been recognized for more than 2000 years. A Chinese official warned people of the danger of crossing from China into Afghanistan because of the high mountains he would have to cross. He called the mountains "the *Headache Mountains* where men's bodies become feverish, they lose color and are attacked with headache and vomiting."[6]

The incidence of acute mountain sickness varies from 9% to as much as 58%. The greater the altitude the greater the risk of the disease.

The illness is characterized by headache, nausea, fatigue, dizziness and insomnia. It begins about 6 hours after arrival at more than 8,000 feet. The symptoms worsen over the next 2-3 days. It can progress to peripheral edema, ataxia, and changes in mental status.

---

[6] Taylor, Andrew, High-Altitude Illnesses: Physiology, risk factors, prevention, and treatment. RMMJ 2011;2(1)e0022

What are the risk factors for getting acute mountain sickness? Sex is not a factor. Men and women are at equal risk for getting sick. Nor does age appear to be important. The main factors are the rate of ascent and the altitude at which you sleep at night. The faster you ascend the mountain the more likely you are to get sick. Travelling from San Antonio to Vale on the same day you start to ski puts you at significant risk. Genetics probably plays a role. Some people are more susceptible than others to getting sick at altitude.

High altitude cerebral edema (HACE) is likely a more severe form of acute mountain sickness. Acute mountain sickness generally abates by the third day at altitude but HACE is often fatal. It is characterized by confusion, headache, ataxia and photophobia. Over time the patient becomes comatose. The diagnosis is established by finding ataxia and altered consciousness in a patient with AMS or high altitude pulmonary edema (HAPE). Most likely, the disease is due to increased permeability of the blood-brain barrier resulting in fluid leaking into the brain causing cerebral edema or swelling of the brain. Treatment is emergent! Immediate descent from altitude is paramount. High dose steroids can be given along with the descent. Many climbing companies carry inflatable hyperbaric chambers to treat HACE in their clients. The disease can be fatal if the brain herniates though rigid channels in the skull, usually the foramen magnum.

High Altitude Pulmonary Edema can be a fatal disease. It is also associated with acute mountain sickness. The patient becomes fatigued and short of breath with a dry cough. Fever may be present as well. The patient breathes rapidly and has a rapid pulse. On examination, basilar crackles are heard. It is more common than believed. In one ski resort at about 7,000 feet altitude, over a period of seven years there were 47 cases. Likely it is caused by hypoxia. The hypoxia causes pulmonary artery vasoconstriction. This causes shifts in the distribution of blood in the lungs. Parts of the lung get too much blood which causes capillary dilatation and leakage of protein into the alveoli as well as alveolar hemorrhage. The key to the treatment is again rapid descent from altitude but oxygen and rest may be helpful as well.

Chronic Mountain Sickness (Monge's disease) is an exaggerated compensation. The hemoglobin levels may increase to up to 28 gm/100cc. Despite this, the patient experiences fatigue, weakness, headache, confusion, hypoxemia, and cyanosis.

Lastly, high altitude worsens sleep apnea. This effect is aggravated by alcohol consumption!

The treatment of high altitude disorders is to return at once to a lower altitude (less than 4000 feet). Oxygen should be used during the descent, but oxygen alone is not enough. **Descent to low altitude is required.**

Pretreatment (prior to ascending to altitude) with Diamox, a carbonic anhydrase inhibitor, may be helpful in preventing acute mountain sickness but the best prevention is avoiding alcohol, getting adequate rest on arriving at altitude, AND IF GOING UP HIGHER THAN 10,000 FEET, ASCEND IN STAGES IN ORDER TO ACCLIMATICIZE.

Youth is **no** guarantee you won't get sick.

Diving

The key to understanding the effects of diving is Boyle's law and the fact that water is not compressible. The deeper you dive, the greater the pressure surrounding your body and hence your lungs. At 33 feet, the atmospheric pressure is doubled, and the lung volume is halved. At 66 feet, the atmospheric pressure is trebled and the lung volume cut to a third. For example, if we dive to 33 feet the atmospheric pressure will double. Using Boyle's Law ($P_1V_1 = P_2V_2$) and assuming a total lung capacity (TLC) of 6 liters at sea level we can calculate the expected TLC:

$$V_2 = (760 \text{ mm} \times 6 \text{ liters})/1520 \text{ mm} = 3 \text{ liters}$$

The other lung volumes are affected as well. If the forced vital capacity is reduced from 4 liters to 2 liters, the limit of our breathing capacity will be exceeded quickly with exertion. Imagine having a vital capacity of 2 liters while exercising strenuously.

Scuba divers can dive to up to 130 feet or a depth equivalent to 5 atmospheres. Thus, without their pressure tanks, their lung volumes would be cut to a fifth, from a total lung capacity of 6 liters to a total lung capacity of 1.2 liters! Their FVC would be decreased to 0.8 liters! But the pressure tanks prevent the loss in lung volumes.

The lung is not the only organ compressed by the change in atmospheric pressure. Any air filled structure will be compressed. This includes the sinuses as well as the Eustachian tubes which run from the nose to the middle ear. Scuba divers must avoid the tendency to breath-holding during descent to avoid creating a large pressure gradient between the middle ear and the nasal passage which could result in a rupture of the tympanic membrane. Diving to more than six feet can actually rupture the tympanic membrane in somebody with sinus disease.

As the diver descends below 90 feet, nitrogen increases in the blood and can cause "nitrogen narcosis", "the rapture of the deep" or the "Martini effect." The diver behaves like he is intoxicated or on a drug like Valium. He might experience a dulling of judgement or become severely confused.

While diving has problems, so does the return to sea level. Rapid ascent from depths greater than 30 feet can result in the bends and also in barotrauma. The "bends" or "decompression sickness occurs because during descent, nitrogen gas moves from the lungs into the tissues. During rapid ascent, the nitrogen gas in the tissues expands and forms bubbles causing pain, and, sometimes even death. The treatment for the "bends" is placing the patient in a hyperbaric chamber and allow a slow ascent or decompression. The second disorder is barotrauma on rapid ascent. The change in pressure can damage the middle ear and the sinuses especially if the patient has sinusitis, an infection or inflammation of the sinuses. Rapid ascent can cause alveolar rupture if the patient has a blocked bronchus. Less commonly, the stomach may even rupture on ascent due to swallowed air. Remember the volume of gas will double from the ascent from just 33 feet. Even scuba divers are at risk. Don't drink a large coke if you are scuba diving!

Man can only dive to about 130 feet but Cuvier Beaked Whales can dive to 10,000 feet or about 300 atmospheres of pressure. Whales are mammals so they have lungs just like us. How is that possible? The whales turn out to have several advantages. Instead of breathing through their mouths, they breathe through blow-holes which are nasal passages located on the top of the whale's head. They have either one or two depending on the species of whale. The blow-holes are surrounded by muscle which can close the hole quite tightly. The respiratory bronchi and bronchioles are reinforced by cartilage. This allows the alveoli to completely collapse when the whales dive to great depths and rapidly expand on ascent. During a dive the whales can use up to 80% of the oxygen in their alveoli while we can only use about 15% of the oxygen in ours. Moreover, the whales have a different form of myoglobin in their muscle cells which bind oxygen better than our myoglobin. Their myoglobin functions as a store for oxygen during prolonged dives which sometimes last up to two hours!

Scuba divers breathe compressed air or a compressed oxygen-helium mixture delivered with a full face mask in order to prevent the problems with lung compression. The compressed air in the tank helps maintain the diver's lung volumes and the full face mask help avoid problems with the nasal passages and sinuses. SCUBA is "self-contained underwater breathing apparatus" and was developed by Cousteau and Gagnan in 1942. The equipment used today was invented by Eldred and first sold as the Porpoise Regulator in 1952.

The most common style of diving is "breath-holding." Certainly this is the most popular form of diving, but it is also the most dangerous! Competitive breath-holding divers are amazing. The record for a breathe hold, as of 2008, is 9 minutes. The record for underwater swimming distance is 244 meters! The maximum diving depth using only fins is 112 meters.[7] How many of us stand at the side of the pier, hyperventilate for a few seconds, or even longer, then dive head long into the pool, lake, or ocean. When we dive, oxygen is consumed, the paO2 falls, while carbon dioxide is produced and the paCO2 rises. It is the level of carbon dioxide that tells us we must ascend at once to get a breath of air. The "breaking point", the point when the receptors tell us we must breathe, is about a paCO2 of 55. If we hyperventilate before diving the stores or carbon dioxide will be reduced, and the paCO2 will not reach the critical level before hypoxia makes us unconscious and we drown.

The flip side of this is the mammalian diving reflex which consists of **bradycardia** and **peripheral vasoconstriction** occurring after a sudden breath-held deep dive. There have been cases of children falling into deep, cold water, and surviving up to forty minutes, likely due to the presence of this reflex. But I would not count on it when you are diving with friends. It is best not to hyperventilate before diving in the water.

Still, "diving" can be helpful. We use hyperbaric chambers to increase the amount of oxygen delivered to the tissues. At sea level there is about 0.3 cc of dissolved oxygen per 100 cc of blood. For every 100 torr increase in the paO2, the dissolved O2 increases by 0.3. At two atmospheres the pAO2 is 200 torr, thus doubling the amount of dissolved oxygen. Hyperbaric therapy increases the amount of oxygen available to the tissues. It is especially helpful in healing wounds due to ischemia (lack of oxygen) as well as wounds due to anaerobic organisms (anaerobic bacteria don't like oxygen), and in treating carbon monoxide gas poisoning by increasing the elimination of the carbon monoxide. Normally the half-life of CO in the blood is 5 hours because of the tight bonding of carbon monoxide to hemoglobin.

---

[7] Levett, DZH and Millar, IL, Bubble trouble: a review of diving physiology and disease, Postgrad Med J; 84:571-8, 2008

One concept about diving that causes some confusion is the CO2-O2 paradox. At great depths the lung volumes decrease and the concentration of CO2 and O2 increase in the alveoli. At a depth of 33 feet, the alveolar O2 is about 200 and the alveolar CO2 is 80. Thus at this depth there is a greater concentration of carbon dioxide in the alveolus than in the blood and carbon dioxide transfers from the alveoli to the capillaries rather than the reverse. On the other hand, over time, the oxygen is transferred from the alveoli to the blood, so that as the diver ascends and the pressure decreases, the alveolar oxygen may become quite low relative to the arterial oxygen. Thus oxygen will move from the blood to the alveoli.

Exercise

Exercise places a great demand upon the lungs, heart, and muscles. The blood flow to the muscles increases twenty five times compared to resting blood flow. At rest the muscles account for 35-40% of the oxygen consumption, while with exercise they may account for as much as 95%. In addition exercising muscles produce heat, up to 20 times the resting level. Lastly oxygen consumption can increase up to twenty times the resting levels.

Sitting quietly, we breathe in and out about six liters of air a minute. When we exercise we increase the amount of oxygen we need as well as the amount of carbon dioxide we produce. Yet we must maintain our blood level of oxygen and carbon dioxide constant. Therefore, during strenuous exercise the minute ventilation can increase up to 20 fold to as much as 120 liters of air a minute and the cardiac output can increase six-fold. The alveolar ventilation can increase to 60% of the maximum voluntary ventilation in fact.

What causes the increased alveolar ventilation we see with exercise? **Despite the increased O2 demand and CO2 production, neither the paO2 nor the paCO2 change.** Most likely the increased alveolar ventilation is due to sensory fibers in the muscles, tendons, and joints sending signals to the respiratory centers in the medulla to increase the ventilation. Increased body temperature may play a role as well. It is possible that the gray matter that tells us to run or bike also tells the respiratory centers to make us breathe deeper and faster.

The increase in ventilation is mainly due to increased tidal volume and not increased breathing rate. However with heavy exercise, the tidal volume may increase to 60% of the vital capacity and the rate of respiration to 30. If the vital capacity is 4 liters then the tidal volume may be 2.4 liters, nearly five times normal. With the onset of exercise, alveolar ventilation increases within a few seconds; then over the next few minutes it slowly increases till it plateaus. When exercise is stopped the alveolar ventilation returns to normal immediately.

Diffusion increases as exercise increases. It may triple in fact. The greater cardiac output results in better matching of ventilation and perfusion in the lung. Because of the increased alveolar ventilation, with increasing amounts of exercise the pAO2 – paO2 gradient actually increases. This effect will also increase diffusion.

When can exercise be too much? At times, exercise can be so demanding that the body may not be able to get enough oxygen to continue on with aerobic metabolism. When that happens, the muscles will begin to produce lactic acid instead of water and carbon dioxide from glucose. At that point the pH will fall. This is the anaerobic threshold. When this occurs, the H+ ions begin to drive ventilation and the ventilation increases faster than oxygen uptake. Thus the oxygen level remains constant while the paCO2 and pH fall.

In summary, at rest the O2 consumption is 250 cc/min and skeletal muscles account for 40% or so. The brain accounts for 25%. With exercise the O2 consumption increases dramatically and the skeletal muscles may account for up to 95% of the O2 consumption. With mild to moderate exercise, the ABG's are normal. When the anaerobic threshold is crossed the pH and pCO2 both fall although the pO2 remains normal.

The heart is the limiting factor in exercise ability. The cardiac output increases dramatically. It may increase 6 to 8 fold! But the cardiac output can only increase so much and **the cardiac output becomes the limiting factor to exercise capacity**. The increase in cardiac output is largely due to an increase in stroke volume and, to lesser extent, the heart rate. There is also increased sympathetic nerve activity which increases the heart rate and the strength of cardiac muscle contraction. The increased sympathetic activity also causes peripheral vasoconstriction. Only the muscles involved in the exercise, the heart itself, and the brain are spared the vasoconstriction.

How do we determine how much to exercise? When is enough, enough? The best way is to look at the maximum heart rate based on age. The maximum heart rate equals 220 minus age in years. Thus at age 20 the maximum is 200 (220-20). At age 70 the maximum is 150 (220-70). Aerobic exercise should be done at 80% of the maximum heart rate. Thus at age 20 you should aim at a heart rate of 160, while at 70 you should aim for 120.

What are the benefits of exercise? The athletic heart is larger and stronger. The mass of the heart may increase up to 40% in marathon runners. The risk of the metabolic syndrome is decreased. In fact, the onset of diabetes can be delayed for years. The LDL or bad cholesterol is reduced. The good cholesterol increases. The bone density is increased. Sleep is better. Energy level is higher. People who exercise have less stress, depression, and anxiety. But, remember weight loss only happens with diet!

Exercise appears to work by both lengthening the telomeres and changing our gene expression. Each of our chromosomes is capped by a sequence of DNA bases called a telomere. The telomere prevents the chromosome from dividing improperly. It works like the plastic tip on your shoelace. Each time the cell divides the telomere shortens until the telomere is so short the cell can no longer divide at all and it dies. The white blood cells in babies have telomeres with more than 8000 base pairs while the elderly have only 2000. Most scientists believe this process is related to aging, cancer and even death though it is likely only one small part of the process. Still, regular exercise lengthens the telomeres!

The second change that daily exercise produces is that it resets our genetic expression to our normal baseline. Not all our genes our expressed all the time. There are gatekeepers that turn on and turn off some of our genes. Sedentary people have genes that are reset to their lifestyle. Their arteries become more constricted and more inflamed. Exercise resets the genes to our healthy baseline and thus improves circulation. The earlier we begin to exercise the better. Better to start as a child but if you are 20, better to start at 20!

There are some potential downsides to exercise. Heat production can increase up to 20 fold and heat stroke may occur. This is more likely in humid conditions and with excess clothing. Weight can drop easily 5-10 lbs. in an hour of exercise due to water loss. The symptoms of heat stroke include a cessation of sweating, nausea, headache and weakness. The patient becomes unsteady on his or her feet and confused. Circulatory collapse may follow and the patient may lapse into coma. Do not run in the heat of the day! Wear appropriate clothes! Be aware of the early symptoms of heat stroke. Take plenty of water but not salt. Stop exercising at once if you feel unwell.

IMPORTANT CONCEPTS TO REMEMBER FROM THIS LECTURE

1. The treatment of high altitude sickness is oxygen?

    False. The patient must be brought down to an altitude of less than 4000 feet

2. At a 130 feet dive (5 atmospheres) the expected total lung capacity is about

    1.2 liters.

3. During strenuous exercise the paO2 falls?

    False

4. What is the limiting factor in how much we can exercise?

    The cardiac output.

Peter A. Petroff, MD

Lecture Twenty-two

Immunology

Every day we are exposed to chemicals, toxins, and microorganisms of all kinds. The viruses, bacteria, and other living creatures we encounter all want to survive. Some of them even need our bodies in order to survive! They consider us a great source of nutrients. We are in a constant battle for survival against many of these invaders. Over the last 500 million years our bodies have developed a complex means of defense called the **mammalian immune system.**

Immunity is the ability to recognize and eliminate foreign invaders from our body. It depends upon the fact that all entities, even normal tissue, have "antigens" which are chemical markers located on the surface of all cells In addition an antigen may be something in the environment, such as chemicals, bacteria, viruses, or pollen. When antigens foreign to our body, even cancer cells which develop inside of us, are found, they are destroyed. However, sometimes the body makes a mistake and identifies normal tissue as a foreign antigen, resulting in an autoimmune disorder such as Rheumatoid Arthritis.

It should be obvious that developing a system of defense is difficult. After all, we depend upon the bacteria in our gut to make some of the vitamins we need and even help us digest our food. In fact, our bodies have more bacteria than cells! We don't want to kill the good bacteria. Thus the requirements of a good defense must be that it will:

- **Attack foreign threats.** The threats from different organisms covers a vast range of physical sizes from toxins less than one nanometer in diameter up to parasitic worms which can be as long as 20 meters in length.

- **Live in harmony with needed bacteria.** The bacteria in our gut are necessary for digesting food and vitamins. They must be protected.

- **Eliminate internal threats.** The system must destroy our damaged cells, some of which may become cancerous.

- **Not cause damage when it functions.** The system must not result in damage to our own healthy tissue.

What is immunology? It is the study of the "Immune System". The word "immune" is from the Greek *immunis* and means **exempt.** The key primary lymphoid organs of the immune system are the **thymus and bone marrow** as well as secondary lymphatic tissues such as the **spleen, tonsils, lymph vessels, lymph nodes, adenoids and skin.** The main components of the immune system are present widely in the circulation throughout the body and not associated with any specific organ.

The first form of immunity was developed billions of years ago. It is called **innate immunity.** It is quick acting but non-specific. It recognizes classes of organisms by identifying key molecules associated with many different types of invaders. All invaders are treated the same. And it can't create a memory of the event. The second type of immunity, **adaptive immunity**, developed five-hundred million years ago and is common to all vertebrates. It is very specific to each target and it creates a memory or history of the invasion and thus is prepared for the next attack by the same or similar invader. Specific antibodies are developed which result in a specific response.

Innate immunity is quite complex and is used by all organisms. It involves three components: barriers, cellular components and chemical components.

Barriers include such things as the unbroken stratum corneum of the skin. The stratum corneum is non-living but it contains sebum, a chemical which produces antibacterial fatty acids. In addition the epidermal cells produce **defensins** which are also antibacterial chemicals.

The respiratory system also has an excellent system of barriers. The mucous membranes of the nose and lungs provide an effective barrier system. The nose traps all particles larger than 10 micra and absorbs soluble gases such as sulfur dioxide. Because of the rapid flow in and out of the nose the particles impact on the wall of the nasal structure making clearance of invaders even more effective. If any invaders get into the lung they impact on the wall of the trachea and bronchi and the mucociliary action sweeps the particles into the throat where they are cleared by coughing.

Examples of the cellular innate immunity include the **Langerhans cells** found in our skin, and **natural killer cells** found in our blood, both of which phagocytize or eat the foreign invaders. Another example of cellular innate defense is the Mast Cell found in the lung which produces histamine. The histamine causes vasodilation increasing the blood flow to the damaged tissue. The Mast Cell also releases leukotrienes which attract phagocytic cells to the area.

Innate lung cellular immunity includes the alveolar macrophages and the lung's own natural killer cells. Alveolar macrophages form the first line of defense against alveolar invaders. They are derived from monocytes in the blood. They act to identify the microbe, engulf it and destroy it. The natural killer cells found in lung tissue activate the alveolar macrophages.

Examples of chemical innate immunity include both Interferon which blocks replication of viruses and Complement which lyses cellular antigens making them more recognizable. In addition there are Lysozymes in our saliva that can destroy bacteria.

There are many innate chemical defenses of the lung. They include chemicals found in the airway secretions such as Lactoferrin which binds iron depriving bacteria of a needed nutrient, Lysozyme which destroys bacterial cell walls and Antitrypsins which protect the lining of the lung from proteases released by bacteria. In addition to these chemicals, the lung also activates the complement system which is the major soluble protein involved in innate immunity. It attracts polymorphonucleocytes (PMN) and coats the bacteria enabling them to be lysed by the macrophages. The alveolar type 2 cell and Club Cell produce Surfactant which contains proteins called Collectins which attract macrophages and have a potent detergent effect to help lyse bacteria. These chemicals are responsible for the inflammatory reaction. Complement produces chemotaxins which attract the polymorphonucleocytes as well as additional macrophages. The polymorphonucleocytes produce superoxide, hydrogen peroxide, and ion radicals which increase their killing power and defensins which are capable of killing fungal organisms

Adaptive Immunity is specific immunity. The key players are the lymphocytes and macrophages. Two types of lymphocytes are involved. The T cells, named after the Thymus gland where they were first found, are produced in the bone marrow and thymus gland. The B cells are produced by the embryonic bone marrow and adult lymph nodes. They are named after the "Bursa of Fabricus" which is a collection of lymph nodes in the gut of embryonic chickens. There are several types of T lymphocytes. The T4 lymphocytes or helper lymphocytes and the T8 or killer lymphocytes are examples.

How does the system work? When a foreign substance is encountered, the macrophages, and to less extent, the T lymphocytes, ingest the substance and expose its antigens. They recognize it as foreign and activate the immune reaction. The T4 lymphocytes or helper cells are activated and some of these cells become memory cells which are permanently sensitized to the antigen. Others are converted into T8 or cytotoxic (killer) lymphocytes which destroy the foreign substance. The T4 cells also produce cytokines which attract even more macrophages to the area. The T4 lymphocytes are important in still another way. The T4 helper lymphocytes stimulate the B lymphocytes to become both memory cells and plasma cells. The plasma cells then secrete antibodies which are specific to the antigen. Thus the T4 cells are the keys to adaptive immunity in that they are involved directly in causing the production of antibody and in developing a memory of the attack. However, it is the B cells which make the antibody. The T lymphocytes do not make antibodies. Lastly when the battle is won, the T4 suppressor cells turn off the reaction so the chemicals released by the macrophages don't destroy the host tissue.

What are antibodies? Antibodies are complex proteins shaped like the letter Y. The antibodies **do not** actually destroy the antigen. Instead they bind to the antigen forming an antibody-antigen complex which effectively marks the antigen-carrying cell, bacteria or virus for destruction which will be carried out by the macrophages. There is ONE and only one kind of antibody for each kind of antigen and the antibodies stay in the memory cells for decades.

There are several types of antibodies. IgA is found in tears, saliva and breast milk. IgG is found in the blood and extracellular fluid. IgM is a large complex immunoglobulin which is important in the early response to infection. It provides the initial immune response to an antigen. IgG then follows later. IgE is found on mast cells and in the gut and is important in allergy as well as in the immune response to parasites. Lastly, IgD is found on receptors on B lymphocytes.

Lastly, there is a type of immune response that involves neither antibodies nor the immune system. Certain genes produce chemicals which prevent the infection. This response is actually programmed in the DNA. That is why dogs and cats are immune to measles, only mice get mouse leukemia (we can't get it from them), and monkeys don't get infected with the HIV virus.

As we age, the immune system ages as well. The elderly are more likely to have a recurrence of the chicken pox virus in the form of Shingles, the elderly are more likely to get infections such as influenza and die from it and they are more likely to get cancer. These are all failures of the the immune system!

Acquired Immunodeficiency Syndrome (AIDS)

In the early 1980's, an unusual infection, Pneumocystis jiroveci, usually found only in immunosuppressed patients following a kidney transplant, began appearing in otherwise healthy young men in Los Angeles. All the young men were homosexual. At nearly the same time, in New York, Kaposi's sarcoma, a very rare tumor, was found in several drug users in New York. It soon became clear that the men had become immune-incompetent due to a viral infection which was transmitted from person to person. In 1983: the virus was isolated from a patient and the following year the Human Immunodeficiency Virus (HIV) was identified as the causative agent of the Acquired Immunodeficiency Syndrome (AIDS). The next year a blood test, an enzyme linked immunosorbent assay or ELISA, was developed and early identification of patients with AIDS could be made.

Where did the virus come from? Most likely it came from non-human primates in West-central Africa. There are wild chimpanzees in southern Cameroon that have a similar infection. With colonization by the European powers, prostitution became quite common. By 1928, 45% of the women of Kinshasa were prostitutes. The earliest case of HIV in a human dates to 1959 in the Congo. However, the vast majority of cases outside of Africa can be traced to a few Haitian men who brought the infection to the USA about a dozen years before the outbreak in 1981. Using genetic sequencing of the virus, Dr. Michael Worobey showed that HIV had spread from Africa to the Caribbean by around 1967, and had arrived in the U.S. by around 1971, first in New York City, and then in San Francisco by 1976. By 1981, the virus had already jumped from coast to coast, and had become genetically diverse.

The virus (HIV) is a RNA retrovirus which means it has ribonucleic acid instead of deoxyribonucleic acid as its genetic material. It also carries the enzyme, Reverse Transcriptase, which allows the virus to replicate using the patient's own DNA. The virus binds to a cell that has a CD4 receptor, such as the T4 lymphocyte, macrophage or certain brain cells. After the virus binds to the CD4 receptor, it fuses to the cell wall and its RNA core is injected into the patient's cell. The virus's Reverse Transcriptase then converts the viral RNA into DNA which becomes part of the patient's DNA. The new DNA then produces the virus' RNA, proteins and enzymes which are assembled in the cytoplasm of the patient's cell into whole virus particles which then explode by the thousands from the infected cell.

The primary mode of transmission of the virus is sexual. The virus is found in seminal fluid in infected men and in the vaginal fluid of infected women. Infected male to uninfected female transmission is eight times more likely to result in transmission than that of infected female to uninfected male. Circumcision offers some protection against transmission. This may be due to the fact that the foreskin contains CD4 cells. Oral sex has a very low transmission rate while the most dangerous form of intercourse is anal intercourse.

A second means of transmission is via blood and blood products, including transplanted tissues. Subcutaneous injection is as efficient as IV injection in transmitting the disease. Between 600,000 and 800,000 health workers are injured with needles or other sharp materials a year in the USA. The risk of transmission from an HIV positive patient is only 0.3%. It is far less than the risk of transmission of hepatitis B. Transmission may occur through mucous membrane exposure or even intact skin if the health care worker has a dermatitis.

The last means of transmission is from an infected mother to an infant. This can occur during labor and delivery (intrapartum), immediately after delivery, or through breast milk.

HIV is never transmitted by casual contact such as kissing or by biting insects. Doris Day never got AIDS from Rock Hudson. Nor can you get AIDS from sitting on a toilet seat or from a mosquito bite.

The average risk of getting AIDS per exposure is as follows:

Exposure	risk of Infection
Blood transfusion	90%
Childbirth	25%
Needle sharing	.67%
Needle stick	.23% (1 in 300)
Anal intercourse	.03 to 4%
Vaginal intercourse	.01 to .38%

AIDS is a worldwide infection. There are about 36 million people living with the virus as well as 1.8 million new infections every year. In Africa alone there are 22.9 million living with the disease and there were 1.2 million deaths in 2010. In fact, Africa accounted for 66% of all the deaths that year due to AIDS. Five percent of the adult African population has the infection. There were also four million people living with AIDS in Asia, half of whom were in India. In contrast there are only 1.1 million Americans, 86,500 Brits and 65,000 Canadians with the infection. An estimated 37,600 Americans became infected in 2014 but between 2008 and 2014 the rate of infection fell 18%! Southern states account for half the cases of newly diagnosed AIDS.

In the USA, in 1994 there were 50,000 deaths due to AIDS but by 2001 only 15,600 deaths. In 2014, there were only 12,333 deaths in patients who had been diagnosed with AIDS. Of those, 6,721 deaths were attributed directly to HIV. There are about 35,000 to 40,000 new cases a year. Half of the infections occur in people less than 25 and two-thirds occur in people less than 40. In 2014 about 1.1 million people were living with HIV. About 20% were unaware of their infection. In fact nearly 40% below the age of 25 were unaware of the diagnosis.

The World Health Organization set 90-90-90 as the goal for 2020. They want 90% of patients infected with the virus to be aware of the infection, 90% to be getting care for the infection, and 90% of those to be virally suppressed. At the present 75% of infected Americans are aware of the infection and only half are virally suppressed.

In the United States there are about 30,000 new cases a year, most of these young adults from 25 to 35 years of age. Gay and bisexual male contact accounted for two thirds of HIV diagnoses while heterosexual male contact accounted for a quarter. Women represented only 19% of cases. Of these, four-fifths of infection was due to heterosexual contact and only about 12% due to drugs. In fact, over all, drug use accounted for only 9% of cases in both men and women. Of new cases Anglos (non-Hispanic whites) account for 31%, Hispanics account for 25% while representing 16% of the population and Blacks account for 42% while accounting for 12% of the population. Asians represent 6% of the population but have only 2% of infections.

The course of illness begins with inoculation of the virus. The symptoms of HIV disease are due to a profound immunodeficiency resulting primarily from a progressive quantitative and qualitative deficiency of helper T cells.

Inoculation most often occurs through sexual transmission. When the virus enters the body it infects the CD4 cells and rapidly replicates inside them. The T8 "killer cells" are activated and kill most of the HIV infected cells. Six weeks after inoculation the patient may have a viral-like syndrome resembling infectious mononucleosis. This phase lasts 1-2 weeks. At this point the blood test will become positive for the HIV infection. This change is called a seroconversion.

A long latent period follows. The virus is continually reproducing, constantly changing its RNA, but the body's immune system is able to keep up. There is a state of generalized immune activation. This phase generally lasts about ten years.

Finally the immune system crashes and the patient develops AIDS. The body is no longer able to keep up and the CD4 count falls and the number of viral particles increases. Pneumonia, especially due to Streptococcus pneumoniae and H. influenza, are common. As the CD4 count falls below 200 per microliter the patient develops an infection such as pneumocystis jiroveci pneumonia or a cancer such as Kaposi's sarcoma. When the count falls still further to below 50, Mycobacterium avium infection occurs. The infection may actually become systemic and even be grown in the blood.

The diagnosis is made through blood testing. There are two tests available for the diagnosis. The first is the ELISA or enzyme immunoassay (EIA) which is 99.5% sensitive but has a 90% false positive in low risk groups. Because of the high rate of false positive, this test should always be confirmed with an antibody tests which measures HIV1, HIV2 and p24 antigens. The Western Blot test is outdated and no longer in use.

In addition, two tests are used to monitor the course of the disease and to help make decisions regarding changes in treatment: the CD4 count and the RNA viral load. The CD4 is the laboratory test accepted as the best indicator of the immediate state of immunologic competence of the HIV infected patient. If it is less than 200, pneumocystis may occur and prophylaxis against that agent should be begun. If it is less than 50, both Cytomegalovirus virus infection and M. avium infection may occur. Prophylaxis against M. avium should begin. The second test, RNA viral load, measures the number of virus in the blood but even when the viral load is undetectable that does not mean there are no viruses!

In the past, various levels of the CD4 count and RNA viral load were used to determine when to treat HIV infection. Now, all patients are treated from the time of the diagnosis.

Prevention is, of course, the best course of treatment. Consistent condom use reduces the risk of transmission by 80%. Circumcision reduces the risk between 38 and 64%, at least in Africa. However the use of a spermicide may increase the risk because of vaginal irritation. Taking antiviral medication prior to risky sex will to a large extent prevent infection. **But sexual abstinence education does not affect HIV risk.**

Treatment is extremely effective. In fact HIV has now become a chronic disease like COPD or CHF rather than an acute and fatal disease. The main problem with therapy for AIDS is that it is extremely expensive, easily exceeding 30,000 dollars a year. How can someone living in poverty afford it?

Without treatment the average survival is 9 to 11 years which is still better than congestive heart failure. With treatment, the young adult can live between 20 and 50 years. If the treatment is begun after the diagnosis of AIDS the outlook is still 10 to 40 years of life. But half of the infants born with HIV die before the age of two.

While HIV infection is the main cause of death, neurocognitive disease, osteoporosis, neuropathy, cancers, renal disease and heart disease often contribute to the patient's death as well. In addition the Epstein Barr Virus causes lymphomas, Herpesvirus 8 causes Kaposi's sarcoma, Hepatitis B and C cause liver cancer, Helicobacter pylori cause stomach cancer and the Papillomavirus causes anogenital cancers. Some patients are even dying of tumors related to the successful therapy of their AIDS. Lung cancer and leukemia are more common in patients with HIV but there isn't any increase in breast, prostate and ovarian cancers.

What about respiratory therapists and the drawing of blood gases? As of 2002, 57 health care workers had become infected with HIV as a result of professional activities, including 19 laboratory workers, 24 nurses, 6 physicians and 1 RT. Most exposures were to blood products. Most were from needle sticks. As of December 31, 2013, there have been 58 confirmed occupational transmissions of HIV and 150 possible transmissions in the United States. Of these, only one confirmed case has been reported since 1999.

If you are stuck by a needle drawing a blood gas, the wound should be cleansed immediately and an antiseptic applied. Treatment should be begun at once with a combination of three anti-HIV agents. This should reduce the risk of HIV infection to nearly zero.

But again, prevention is the key! Not all HIV infected patients are known. Treat all patients as if they are infected! Always wear gloves when you might be exposed to body fluids and wash your hands after you remove the gloves.

Never recap needles by hand. Always place needles in a puncture resistant container. Keep disposable resuscitation equipment nearby. Health workers with severe dermatitis should not handle patient care materials.

A word must be said about Pneumocystis jiroveci or Pneumocystis carinii (old nomenclature) infection because the respiratory therapist will often be called upon to give prophylactic treatments for prevention of the disease. The organism is a yeast-like fungus or a protozoan or a hybrid of the two types of organisms. It infects only patients who are immuno-incompetent such as transplant patients on immunosuppressive agents or patients with AIDS. The fungus is ubiquitous and worldwide. Most children age 3-4 have been infected by the organism and recovered.

In the patient with AIDS, Pneumocystis jiroveci generally causes a pneumonia which has many different manifestations. The pneumonia may be lobar or multilobar or diffuse. It may be associated with a pneumothorax or collapsed lung. The hallmark of the illness is that there is progressive shortness of breath, with cough and fever. The dyspnea almost always precedes the cough and fever. The diagnosis is made from an induced sputum or bronchial washing smear although a lung biopsy may be necessary at times. The treatment is high dose sulfa drugs such as Bactrim or pentamidine.

More recently pre-exposure prophylaxis (PrEP) to prevent infection with the HIV virus in discordant couples in which one of the couple has the virus while the other does not. The person infected is begun on regular antiviral therapy while the non-infected person is begun on PrEP. The use of PrEP has reduced the rate of infection by 75%. Condoms should also be used.

Who should be tested for HIV? The United States Preventive Services Task Force recommended testing everyone from the age of 13 to 65 but the cost could be prohibitive. At the present time, any patient who has more than one sexual partner or is using intravenous recreational drugs should be tested.

IMPORTANT CONCEPTS TO REMEMBER FROM THIS LECTURE

1. Immunity is defined as:

    The ability to recognize and eliminate foreign invaders from the organism

2. The two types of lymphocytes involved in adaptive immunity are:

    The B and T cells

3. The lymphocytes that are attacked by the HIV virus are the:

    T4 or helper lymphocyte

4. The HIV virus is an:

    RNA virus

INDEX

acetyl choline, 124, 127, 128, 142, 150, 153, 154, 168
acquired immunodeficiency syndrome, 209
Acquired Immunodeficiency Syndrome, 20
Action Potential, 28
acute mountain sickness, 199, 200
Acute Respiratory Distress Syndrome, 97, 98, 112
adaptive immunity, 207
Adaptive Immunity, 208
adenosine, 8, 38, 127
adenosine triphosphate, 21
Adenosine triphosphate, 8
Adenyl Cyclase, 9
aldosterone, 182
allergens, 20
Alveolar Gas Equation, 114
alveolar macrophages, 19, 90
alveolar ventilation, 102, 105, 107, 108, 113, 199, 203
alveolus, 87, 89
Anemia, 13, 14, 18
angina, 39, 41, 50
angiotensin, 182, 184
Angiotensin Converting Enzyme, 51, 182
Antidiuretic Hormone, 181
antigen, 20, 142, 152, 206, 208
aortic, 23, 24
Aortic Stenosis, 26, 52
aortic valve, 23, 24, 27
aortic valve stenosis, 51
Apgar Score, 193
Apnea, 64, 102
Apneustic Center, 130
ARDS, 97, 112
arytenoid cartilages, 69, 70, 73
asbestosis, 149, 154
aspiration, 71, 73
asthma, 12, 18, 20, 52, 67, 73, 102, 105, 107, 117, 124
ATP, 8, 9, 10, 12, 21
atrial fibrillation, 40, 41
Atrial fibrillation, 40, 45
atrial flutter, 39
Atrial Flutter, 39, 40

atrial natriuretic peptide, 182
Atrial Septal Defects, 193
autoimmune disorder, 73, 153, 206
autonomic nervous system, 57, 91, 127
B cells, 20, 208
Bagassosis, 157
basophil, 19
basophils, 19, 20
Biot's Respiration, 103, 104
Bohr Effect, 16
Bohr Equation, 107, 108
Bowman's capsule, 179, 180, 181
Boyle's law, 93, 122, 123, 126
bronchiectasis, 107
Bronchiectasis, 134, 144
Brownian motion, 110
Byssinosis, 157
chemoreceptors, 130, 133
Cheyne-Stokes, 103
Cheyne-Stokes respiration, 176
Coarctation of the Aorta, 54
Collectins, 208
complement, 207
Complement, 207
compliance, 93, 94, 95, 96, 97, 99, 101, 104, 105, 117, 118
congestive heart failure, 18, 37, 47, 50, 51, 63, 64, 83, 103
coronary artery disease, 41, 49
Coronary artery disease, 49, 50
Covalent Bond, 4
cricoid cartilage, 71, 74, 86
cricothyroid membrane, 71
Cyclic AMP, 9
cystic fibrosis, 137, 144
Dalton's law, 113
Deflation Reflex, 131
depolarization, 29
diaphragm, 23, 25, 57, 80, 81, 83, 85, 92, 93, 96, 128, 131
diastole, 25, 27, 32, 47, 48, 50, 51, 55, 56
diffusion, 28, 87, 89
Diphtheria, 72
dorsal respiratory center, 129

Ductus Arteriosus, 54, 128, 193
Eisenmenger's Syndrome., 54
electro-mechanical dissociation, 43
emphysema, 20, 93, 97, 102, 105, 107, 117, 124, 126
encephalitis lethargica, 167
endocardium, 26
Endothelial Reticulum, 2
eosinophil, 19, 20, 22
epiglottis, 66, 69, 70, 71, 73
Epiglottitis, 73
Erythropoietin, 12
Extrinsic Allergic Alveolitis, 157
Farmer's Lung, 157, 158
Fatal familial insomnia, 167
FEV1/FVC ratio, 119, 125, 140
Fick's equation, 112
flow-volume loop, 120
Foramen Ovale, 192, 193
Functional Residual Capacity, 96, 97, 117
Funnel Chest, 79
glomerulus, 179, 181, 183, 184
Graham's law, 111
granulocytes, 18, 19
guanosine cyclase, 143
Head's Paradoxical Reflex, 193
helper lymphocytes, 20
Hematocrit, 13
hemoglobin, 5, 12, 13, 14, 15, 16, 17, 18, 22
Hemoglobin, 4, 13, 14, 15, 16
Hemoglobin concentration, 13
Henderson-Hasselbach, 187
Henderson-Hasselbach equation, 187
Henry's law, 111
Hering-Breuer Reflex, 130, 131
Herring Breuer reflex, 193
High altitude cerebral edema, 200
high altitude pulmonary edema, 200
hippocampus, 129, 165, 166
histamines, 20, 107, 141, 142, 143
Histotoxic Hypoxia, 18
Hot Tub Lung, 157
Human Immunodeficiency Virus, 209
Hyaline Membrane Disease, 98, 194
hyperbaric chambers, 202
hypersensitivity pneumonitis, 155
hypertension, 47, 49
hypocretin, 167, 176

immunity, 20, 206, 207, 208, 213
Immunity, 206, 213
immunology, 206
innate immunity, 206, 207
insomnia, 167, 171
intercostal muscles, 79, 80, 81, 92, 128
Interferon, 207
interstitial lung disease, 124, 154, 155
Ionic Bond, 4
Irritant Reflex, 131, 193
Krebs Cycle, 9
Kulchinsky, 88, 91, 190, 197
Kussmaul's respiration, 103
Lactoferrin, 207
Langerhans, 207
Laplace's Law, 98, 99
larynx, 66, 67, 68, 69, 70, 71, 73
Leucocytes, 18
leukotrienes, 8, 20, 141, 143
Loop of Henle, 179, 181
lymphocyte, 19, 20
Lysosomes, 2
macrophage, 19, 90
Marfan's Syndrome, 53
Mast cells, 20
mediastinum, 19, 24
medulla, 58, 71, 128, 129
Melanoma, 77
Methacholine, 124, 125, 142
mid-maximal flow rate, 119
Mitochondria, 2
mitral, 23, 24
mitral regurgitation, 52
mitral valve, 23, 24, 27
mitral valve prolapse, 52
monocyte, 19
Multifocal Atrial Tachycardia, 41, 45
narcolepsy, 173, 174, 176
natural killer cells, 207
nephron, 179, 183, 186
nephrotic syndrome, 183
Neural crest, 190
non-REM, 165, 166
Non-specific interstitial pneumonitis-fibrosis, 157
notochord, 89
nucleotide, 8
Olfactory Nerve, 67
osmotic pressure, 61, 65, 181, 183

Oxygen, 1, 3, 4, 5, 7, 9, 10, 11, 12, 13, 14, 15, 16, 17, 18
paroxysmal atrial tachycardia, 38
pericardium, 24, 27
Pericardium, 25
pigeon breast, 79
Plasma, 11, 12, 20
Plasma Cells, 20
Platelets, 21
pleura, 79, 81, 82, 83, 88, 91, 131
Pleural effusions, 82
Pneumocystis, 209, 213
Pneumotaxic Center, 130
pneumothorax, 81, 82
Poiseuille's law, 59, 60, 101, 104
poliomyelitis, 152
Polycythemia, 13, 14
Pons, 130
premature atrial contraction, 37
pseudostratified ciliated columnar epithelium, 67, 71, 74
pulmonary embolism, 40, 41, 62, 63, 64
Pulmonary Embolism, 62
pulmonary fibrosis, 53, 93, 102, 105, 112, 117, 126
pulmonary stenosis, 24
pulmonary valve, 24
pulmonic valve, 23, 27
Red Blood Cell, 11, 12
REM sleep, 165, 166
renin-angiotensin-aldosterone system, 182
Residual Volume, 117, 118
Respiratory Distress Syndrome, 98, 194
retrovirus, 209
Reverse Transcriptase, 209
Ribosomes, 2
Sarcoidosis, 64, 149, 155, 159, 160
serotonin, 20, 131
Serum, 11, 12
shingles, 76, 77

Silicosis, 149, 155, 163
Sinus arrhythmia, 37
sinusitis, 67, 68, 72
sleep, 1, 10, 68, 164, 165, 166
smell, 67, 68
Speech, 71
spirogram, 118
squamous epithelium, 67
Starling's Law, 60, 61
sternum, 23, 24
suppresser lymphocytes, 20
surface tension, 90, 97, 98
surfactant, 90, 91, 97, 98
Surfactant, 90, 97, 98, 190, 194, 208
Swallowing, 71
systole, 26, 27, 32, 47, 49, 50, 51, 52, 56
T cells, 20, 208, 211, 213
taste, 67, 68
Tetralogy of Fallot, 53, 54
thrombocytes, 21
Thrush, 73
Thymus Gland, 24
thyroid cartilage, 69, 70
Tidal Volume, 117
total lung capacity, 117
Transposition of the Great Vessels, 54
tricuspid, 23
tricuspid valve, 23, 27
Trigeminal Reflex, 193
usual interstitial pneumonitis, 154, 156
uvulopalatopharyngoplasty, 68
Van Der Waals Bond, 4
Velcro Rales, 154, 155
Vena Cava, 24
ventral respiratory center, 129
ventricle, 24
ventricular arrhythmias, 42
vocal cords, 69, 70, 71, 73, 128
Zyrem, 177

Made in the USA
San Bernardino, CA
21 August 2019